Developmental Group Work
with Adolescents

Developmental Group Work
with Adolescents

Leslie Button

A HALSTED PRESS BOOK

John Wiley & Sons
New York

Published in the U.S.A.
by Halsted Press, a Division of
John Wiley & Sons, Inc.
New York

Library of Congress Cataloging in Publication Data

Button, Leslie.
  Developmental group work with adolescents.

  'A Halsted Press book.'
  Includes bibliographical references and index.
  1. Group relations training.   2. Adolescence.
  I. Title.

HM134.B88   1975   301.18'5   74–26787
ISBN 0–470–12775–9

Printed in Great Britain

To my wife

Contents

Figures

Preface

It is appropriate that a book on group work should be the outcome of the collaborative efforts of a number of people, and in writing this book I should like to pay tribute to the large team of people who have contributed to the long-term programme of exploration and experiment upon which it is based. The use of 'we' in the text that follows has very real significance, for it is used to denote a growing fraternity of workers, who have both contributed to and drawn from the framework upon which this book is based.

Successive generations of trainees following the full-time courses for youth workers and teachers at the University College of Swansea have each helped to deepen our knowledge and insights, and have added to the techniques and skills at our disposal. Teams of tutors in various parts of the country have added a distinctive contribution through a series of experiments in in-service training, and the very large number of trainees engaged in that in-service training have been at the core of the experiments and experience. We have reason to be grateful also to the very large number of young people who have responded to our approaches and have helped us, often consciously, to increase our expertise.

Our approach throughout has been pragmatic. Sometimes it has been inspired in advance by theoretical thinking, but more often the framework of concepts has been evolved out of repeated experience rather than the reverse. The purpose of the programme has been to develop techniques and to evolve a rationale that will make our work more effective, and will contribute to group work as an expertise. Experiment in method and the spirit of group work are as one, and what follows is offered as a contribution to the ever-moving explorations of how we can help one another live full and satisfying lives in a world of rapid change.

The book is first about developmental group work, but since so much of our experience has been with adolescent groups, the weight of attention is inevitably in that direction. However, the range of groups has been much wider, and the same approaches have been used in work with adult groups, notably with groups of teachers, youth workers, and other professional in-service training groups. It is clear that through group work we can help so many people improve their quality of life. Some need only to see more clearly the alternatives open to them, but others need support and encouragement when experimenting with new approaches to life. Many young people are at a specially flexible time of life, but growth and development is open to us all, young and old alike.

CHAPTER ONE

Introduction

The meaning of group work

If you were asked to describe yourself how would you reply? Would you first refer to your formal functions in life, as teacher, youth worker, student, social worker, or would you turn to your more personal roles: father of three, a wife, John's fiancée? If the question were changed to 'What kind of person are you?', would you again answer in terms of contact with other people: 'I'm an easy going sort', or 'I am quite sociable', or 'I keep myself to myself'? When describing other people, the response may be even more directly in terms of their behaviour, and their approach and response to other people. Even our names conjure up in us a whole framework of family connections.

To be human is synonymous with being in communication and in relationship with other people, which demands of us a range of social skills. In accommodating ourselves to other people we will also have to accept some of their demands upon us, which, together with our natural concern for them, is the source of much of their influence upon us. Even when we are at our solitary pursuits, we may be looking over our shoulder to see the reaction of the people around us.

Thus our personal satisfaction, growth and development is achieved mainly through the part that we play in the lives of other people and they in ours. Group work is about helping people in their growth and development, in their social skills, in their personal resource, and in the kind of relationships they establish with other people. Social skills can be learnt only in contact with other people, and it is the purpose of group work to provide the individual with opportunities to relate to others in a supportive atmosphere, to try new approaches and to experiment in new roles. The health of the wider community also will depend on the individual's social skill, and his empathy with and his concern for others.

The individual has to cope with a whole range of relationships which are very different one from another. Although he has experienced a child–parent relationship, he must also achieve a satisfactory parent–child relationship when his turn comes. He must be able to cope with authority as well as with equal or peer relationships, and with relationships which bring conflict as well as easy and supportive ones. Much group work is focussed on peer relationships, especially the give-and-take with intimate equals which is particularly relevant to the adolescent.

The group worker will try to help the group and the individuals within it to work out their own destiny. The relationships between the members of the group and the social controls embedded within the group will be important instruments of development. The group worker will be involved in deliberate action, which implies that he must be well informed about the dynamics of groups, have recourse to a repertoire of techniques, and be skilled in using them.

The range of group work

Although the term 'group work' is reserved for those who are knowingly working through groups for the benefit of the people involved in them, there are many others who stand in a leadership role to groups of people, and are, as it were, unself-conscious group workers. Whether they be teachers, youth workers, clergy, industrial managers, or workshop foremen, at every turn they are having an effect on the people they lead, and on the way in which groups of people influence one another. They too, are themselves caught up in the pattern of relationships and controls of the groups that they lead. It is not a question of whether these people *wish* to influence, often in a very personal way, those whom they lead, but rather *how* they influence them. In many cases their leadership could be much more beneficial if they were more aware of the social processes that surround them, and some of the skills of the group worker can be carried into many other walks of life.

Within the field of work that is recognised as deliberate group work there are a number of branches. The setting within which the work is carried on has a considerable influence on both the purpose and style of work, as, for example, in a school, at a youth club, in the street, in prison, or in a mental hospital. Whilst it is with small groups that most of the more personal work is attempted, it is not always appreciated that the person who is working with larger groups is equally a group worker, though possibly of a different kind. In this book I shall be referring to him as the institutional group worker. By 'institution' I mean the more complex establishment, with a recognised membership, that exists for the help, guidance, or development of its members. The range of such institutions is wide: the youth club, the recreative centre, the school, the church, and the therapeutic community to name only a few.[1]

Although the institutional worker may not be dealing with the same kind of face-to-face situations as in work with small groups, many of the same forces are at work. The individuals and small groups within the larger establishment will be influenced by what takes place in the group as a whole, including the overall climate, the pattern of association and interaction, and the social controls attached to the larger group. In many cases the impact is accidental—though no less inevitable or powerful—and it is questionable whether anything so accidental can be classed as group work at all. It is most important that work of this kind should be seen in its full complexity, especially since it is so often justified in terms of the opportunities for personal experience provided by the association and relationship between the participants.

It would be possible also to classify group work by its particular purpose, which can differ greatly from therapeutic work with mental patients at one extreme, to, at the other, the support of some objective seen as of benefit to the participants, such as their education, their religious devotion, or their recreation and sport. In between these extremes there is work intended to help the individual in his personal growth and adjustment, which I am calling developmental group work, which in turn shades into recreative group work, concerned with personal extension through activity and companionship.

There are basic areas of knowledge and of skill running through all kinds of group work. A common area of knowledge includes the dynamics of groups, the psychology of personality,

[1] Rapoport, R. N. (1960) *Community as Doctor*. London: Tavistock Press. Konopka, G. (1954) *Group Work in the Institution*. New York: Whiteside.

and the meaning of activity in terms of individual experience. There are also particular areas of knowledge suggested by any special purpose of the work. For example, for therapeutic work a deeper understanding of personality and psycho-pathology is needed; for work intended to encourage the participants to acquire the skills of certain activities some real sophistication in those activities will be necessary; and the worker responsible for a recreative centre must have a good grasp of the personal and social effects of various activities, as well as some knowledge of the processes and disciplines of those activities. Similarly with the skills of group work: there are some basic skills common to most forms of group work, and there are some special skills attached to work designed for specific classes of people. Whether it be for adolescents, for old people, for young children, for lonely house-wives, for prisoners, or for mental patients, there will be a special body of knowledge and certain skills appropriate to that special field of work.

The emphasis

I do not wish to make too much of the various departments of group work, because it would be equally valid to point to the very large area of common ground between them. Indeed, progress in the field of group work could easily be held back by too many divisions growing up, with the result that people working in different, though related, fields fail to learn from one another. This book is therefore first about group work, and subsidiary to this there is an emphasis upon developmental group work with young people crossing the threshold from childhood to adult life. Ottaway, who conducted informal group sessions within a university extramural programme, called his work 'the normal man's therapy', and this would be an apt description of a good deal of developmental group work.[1]

It would be wrong, indeed impossible, to keep developmental group work within closely prescribed limits. Quite spontaneously the group will move into what might be regarded as social therapy, and the spring for this may have been in some fairly specialist activity that had its own body of knowledge and

[1] Ottaway, A. K. C. (1966) *Learning Through Group Experience*. London: Routledge and Kegan Paul.

discipline. It is possible to distinguish between problem or crisis-centred work and developmental work, although the two inevitably flow into one another. Developmental work is especially concerned with building the social competence of the individual so that he becomes more capable of dealing with his own problems.[1]

The fact that the worker will be encouraging self-reliance and self-discovery in the participants demands sound knowledge on his part, in the same way as the teacher who works through discovery rather than didactic methods will need to be even more at home with his subjects. For example, the worker will be leading his groups into an examination of their feelings towards authority and the nature of authority, and into an exploration of friendship, of loneliness, and of a wide range of other relationships. Some will examine sexual relationships and feelings, and may need basic information about sex, and others will be concerned with parents and family, their own childhood and themselves. In order to lead this kind of excursion the worker must have a fund of appropriate knowledge and a sound understanding of the processes involved.

[1] For a fuller examination of this distinction, see page 121.

CHAPTER TWO

Meeting personal need

There is always a tendency for the group worker, teacher, or youth worker to focus upon the overt behaviour of young people as the matter for treatment, whereas the overt behaviour may be only a symptom of underlying causes. We need to be very conscious of the basic springs of behaviour. I have already suggested that the quality of being human may be expressed in terms of the other people in our lives, and many of our basic emotional needs are bound up with our contact with other people.[1] There is, of course, a range of physical needs (for example, for food, shelter, and defence) that seem independent of the people around us, but even the satisfaction of these needs leads us immediately to some form of social organisation. The physical need for sex floods over into a complex mesh of love and affection, and in general our physical needs may include a need for actual bodily contact. Physical contact is important to a baby's growth and development, and it has been argued that the physical stroking of the child is replaced in later life by the more sophisticated forms of social grooming through conversation and other means of communication.[2] It is likely that the need for actual physical contact never leaves most of us completely, though the social mores of our community may block its natural expression.

Companionship

The needs that we have for one another form the basis for social cohesion, and central to them all is the need for companionship

---

[1] For a brief account of human needs, see Fleming, C. M. (1963) *Adolescence: its Social Psychology* (2nd edition, revised). London: Routledge and Kegan Paul. (Chapter 5.)

[2] Bern, E. (1964) *Games People Play*. Harmondsworth: Penguin Books. (Pages 13–14.)

and affection. In our studies of adolescent friendships, young people have demonstrated that the pattern of their affiliative relationships may be very complex. They have helped us to distinguish several levels of companionship, and each of these levels seems to have its own importance. I shall be developing this topic below, and it may suffice at this stage to say that we appear to satisfy our total affiliative need through a combination of relationships at various levels.[1]

There is considerable difference from one person to another in the kind of combination achieved, and it would appear that this is more than an accident of the moment. We each tend to have our characteristic style of relationships. Although the need both to love and to be loved seems basic to most people's fulfilment, there are a few people who seem content without close friends. But very few of the young people without friends whom we have met during research or group work have been satisfied with their position. The satisfaction of the need for friendship demands certain social skills, and too often we have met the vicious circle of those in the greatest need of companionship having the least ability to satisfy that need.[2]

There are different qualities attaching to the various forms of relationships. For example, although the child–parent relationship will be conditioned by individual personalities and circumstances, it has a number of recurring features. There is usually some intimacy within the relationship, which will vary from family to family, and will be affected by the advancing age of the child. It is usually characterised by concern and protectiveness on the part of the parents, which may be prolonged at a level inappropriate to the older child. The element of authority in the relationship, which is sometimes quite strong, often causes trouble between the parent and the older adolescent, notwithstanding the fact that it may be prompted by the parents' continuing concern for the child.

Their feelings towards people in authority loom large in the life of many young people. In many cases they are endeavouring to establish their own autonomy in a reasonable way, but in some there is a blind rejection of, or rebelliousness towards, every person seen as an authority figure. Not all adults will be seen as in

[1] Page 49.
[2] For some discussion about how we might help such people, see page 111.

authority and a distinction must be drawn between attitudes towards authority and attitudes to adults in general. Many youngsters, including some who find it difficult to confide in their peers, can and do accept a friendly adult as a confidant. The confidant relationship should not be confused with friendship: friendship implies an equal and reciprocal relationship, while the confidant may be a recipient only, and a person who is passing the confidences is not required to accept confidences in return. We have found that many of the young people who have difficulty in making friendships can nonetheless establish a relationship with a confidant, generally someone older than himself.

The child–parent and peer relationships

In his early years the child is very dependent on the parent, not only for his physical needs but also for much of his social containment, and it has been customary to lay great stress on the child–parent relationship.[1] There is no doubt that this early relationship will build a great deal into the personality of the child, but as the child becomes older, the basis of his total containment becomes much wider, and the peer relationship assumes greater importance. Indeed, in the years when the youngster is breaking away from the dependence on parents and home, the peer relationship often assumes a dominant position, a tendency which has been reinforced by changes in the broader culture of the community and the creation of a teenage cult.

Yet it has become evident to us in our research that the peer relationship, particularly at an intimate level, is one of the toughest relationships to establish. We have found that so many of the youngsters who consider themselves to be unequal to life, or who are discontented, or delinquent, are in difficulties with their relationships with peers. Some of them experience an easy relationship with their parents, and most can relate readily to an adult confidant, as they do to us in our research or group work. Many teachers and youth workers have been very surprised by sociometric studies which have revealed that the youngster who related to them with so much poise was at odds with his peers. We have met this so frequently that it is customary for us to ask

[1] Bowlby, J. (1966) *Child Care and the Growth of Love.* Harmondsworth: Penguin Books.

ourselves questions about any youngster who is especially amenable or helpful to the adult in, say the classroom or club. Is he seeking a relationship with an adult as a compensation for a lack of firm relationships with peers?

It may be argued that the source of the difficulty that a young person is experiencing with his peers stems from deeper personality factors laid down by the early child–parent relationships, and this may well be true. But by later adolescence the family situation has usually had its effect, and its influence is embedded in the personality of the youngster who is now moving as an independent being. He may be suffering situational difficulties in his home—and some youngsters have to cope with incredible social and physical problems at home[1]—but we shall need to approach him as a person of growing independence, not just as a child locked in a relationship with his parents.

There is an element of continuing social therapy within close friendship, and often real support may be drawn also from a wider circle of companions. Young people who are firmly contained in a warm peer structure may weather many difficult passages at home and in other walks of life; and the peer situation may offer an arena for new roles and experience, or serve as a support when the youngster ventures into new experiences. Unfortunately, some peer situations act in reverse of all this, and will call for the attention of the group worker, as described later in this book.

It is a new thought to many who serve young people professionally that not only the most important but also the most difficult relationship for many adolescents is the intimate relationship with peers. In school an improvement in social conditions is so often seen in terms of the relationship between the teacher and individual child, whereas often the teacher might best serve the child by acting as a catalyst in his forming relationships with peers. Similarly, many youth workers see their pastoral work as striking a friendly or confidant relationship with individual members, whereas they might enable young people to help one another much more effectively than they can help them personally.

---

[1] Clegg, A. and Megson, B. (1968) *Children in Distress*. Harmondsworth: Penguin Books; Schools Council (1970) Working Paper 27, *Cross'd with Adversity: the education of socially disadvantaged children in secondary schools*. London: Evans/Methuen Educational.

Sexual relationships

In many adolescents there is a preoccupation with the sexual relationship. With most, sex is a matter of interest, and for some it is all-absorbing. Sexual experimentation is a normal part of adolescence, and some young people complete their mating and move into married life within late adolescence. In our own studies we have been very interested in the interconnection between friendship and the sexual relationship. There is a good deal of intimacy involved in both these relationships and it is tempting to see one as naturally contained within the other. But many young people have demonstrated to us that they can keep these two relationships apart, for not infrequently young people have insisted that the person with whom they were connected sexually was not a close friend in the sense of the usual intimacies of friendship. Some have insisted that their sexual partner was not a friend at all, but more of a sexual associate, in spite of the fact that the sexual experience was deep and moving, even all-pervading. Some young people have shown themselves as having been engaged to be married to a sexual partner rather than a close friend, and there is reason to believe that a similar kind of relationship may be continued into marriage.

It seems therefore that it is possible to distinguish between love-sex and love-friendship, and that the two may coalesce or they may be kept apart. Some people who are unable to establish deep friendships are able to engage in a sexual relationship, and in this way the sexual relationship serves them very well, for it is possible that they may be able to reach a deeper level of friendship as a result of being drawn to somebody through a sexual relationship. It is as if sex has a functional or task element that makes it different from friendship operating at a highly personal level.

It may be surprising that these two relationships can be handled separately in this Western world of romantic love, but it could be argued that we are asking a great deal when we vest the two relationships in the same person. It is not so in every community. In some communities the marriage is clearly a love-sex relationship, for house-keeping and procreation, and the love-friendship is maintained outside the marriage with peers of the same sex.[1]

[1] For an example of such a community, Stirling, P. (1965) *Turkish Village.* London: Weidenfeld and Nicolson.

Need for significance

We are influenced in much of our behaviour by the need to matter, to be somebody, to have significance. Much of that significance comes from the reflections of ourselves that we see in the eyes of other people, and is therefore bound up with the relationship with other people discussed above. However, some of our relationships may reduce us rather than raise our status.

A need for significance enters our job-seeking, our sport, and our competitive roles. The role that we occupy in life and the status that goes with it play their part, and young people who are at an in-between stage, between childhood and adulthood, may well lend their support to a youth culture with which they can identify. At its most elementary, young people prefer to be noticed rather than be overlooked, and may even lend themselves to mischief in order to gain some attention; many would rather be well hated than not noticed at all. This undoubtedly inspires some of the mischief that takes place in school, and the vandalism that is all too general.

I have been impressed by the clarity with which this has been expressed by a number of the violent groups of youngsters with whom we have been in contact. Formerly, they have explained, they were failures, many of them unhappy at home, spurned by the representatives of the community—often associated in their minds with teachers—and even cowards in their own eyes. Now they experienced warmth and loyalty within their group, had demonstrated their capacity in pitched battles with rival gangs and police, were certainly to be reckoned with by the adult community, and were a thorn in the side of those in authority. And they demonstrated each day that they were not cowards. They clearly felt that they were achieving a degree of self-fulfilment that the normal run of life had denied them.

The need for significance is bound up with our self-concepts, to which I will return in Chapter 6. To put the other person in the position where he matters is one of the basic skills of the group worker, or, for that matter, for anyone who must encourage the efforts of other people.

The need for security

Quite a lot has been made of the effect of insecurity, for example, in the literature about delinquency. To some extent we are saying again that we need companionship, and need to be assured of a place in other people's lives, and that if we are unsure of this then we are insecure. We like to know where we are; doubt and uncertainty can be very exacting. In a television series Hans Hanz postulated that there is a basic human need for order. He illustrated this visually by the way we marshal ourselves in all kinds of situations, and suggested that a need for order permeates every corner of life. Above all, we like to know where we are with other people. This can be seen very clearly in the T-group situation, where roles change quickly and there is no accepted long-term structure of roles and hierarchy.[1] It is particularly uncomfortable for the participants not to know where they stand with the 'consultant', whom they see as an inactive authority figure, behaving in an unexpected way. The group worker may provoke similar feelings if he works through indefinite and unstructured situations. In larger group situations the uncertainty produced by enigmatic leadership can even give rise to sudden flashes of destructiveness.

It is of interest to the group worker that different people seem to have quite different levels of resilience to uncertainty, and there is reason to believe that most of us can learn to develop greater resilience, although the scope for movement may be very different from one person to another. In developing resilience to uncertainty the individual may need help and support, and this is often one of the valid objectives of a particular piece of group work.

Need for adventure and new experience

It may seem a paradox to set the need for adventure and new experience in juxtaposition with the need for security and order. Yet it may reasonably be advanced that a part of that very security is the continuing opportunity to break new ground. What do we mean when we say that we are bored? It surely means that we are caught up in static or repetitive situations, and that we are no longer extending the edges of our experience. Although some of this new experience may be through impersonal events and physical things, much of it will come through our being involved in other people's lives. Many of us endeavour to

[1] See page 67.

satisfy our need largely through vicarious experience offered to us by newspapers, radio and television, as well as through literature and other art forms.

The satisfaction of this need does not turn only on having the opportunity: as with the satisfaction of other needs, such as the need for companionship, we must have the personal capacity to seek our own satisfaction. It means that we must be able to stir ourselves, take action with sufficient effort and persistence for us to derive satisfaction from the opportunities that present themselves. Boredom is an attribute of the person as much as it is of his situation. Young people should be at the peak of their power and freedom in this respect, yet we meet all too many whose curiosity and sense of adventure seem to have been replaced by apathy, timidity and ennui. It tends to be the apathetic who complain most about being bored, and it is sometimes difficult to break through this vicious circle. How far have we been responsible for this through our education system? Has their education fed young people's curiosity or dulled it, prepared them for independence and exploration, or merely inculcated a need for direction?

The same attributes of daring, effort and persistence enter many aspects of life, so that lack of satisfaction is likely to be compounded. It is difficult for us to gain status, and therefore personal significance, in other people's eyes unless we make an effort to do so. Even friendship may be difficult for those who lack the persistence that would make their friendship worth while, or the initiative and effort to respond to the needs of other people.

The needs of the group worker

It would be a mistake when considering the emotional needs of other people, not, at the same time, to be conscious of our own needs. How far are we responding to our own needs when serving as group workers? At a minimum, we are both earning our keep and achieving a certain status. We might even develop a sense of empire, or try to boost our own importance at the expense of other related workers and services. The need for status and the gratification of self-importance is as applicable to the part-time or voluntary worker as to the professional; in fact, the vested interest of the volunteer is sometimes more jealously guarded than that of the professional.

We need to admit to ourselves the satisfactions we derive from our work. We may be doing it because we enjoy responding to the needs of others, or because we find people interesting, and the fact that we can help them and play a part in their lives may give us a sense of importance. These are all valid satisfactions to be derived from a demanding job. Danger arises either from our being unaware of our own needs and the part that they are playing in our work, or from our being so strongly compelled by our own needs that they unduly influence the direction of our work. In this case the young people may be less at the centre of our work than they should be.

It is important that the opportunity, indeed the necessity, for self-assessment should be structured into our work. Ideally this would be provided by a system of supervision, but for much of the time we are likely to be working on our own, and a discipline of recording, planning and preparation will be required to help safeguard us against our own excesses. This discipline of self-assessment will also need to be structured into the initial training or any in-service training of the group worker.[1]

Adolescence

The justification for the emphasis in this book on work with adolescents resides in the nature of adolescence. The family is sometimes described as the womb of society, in which case adolescence represents the birth of the independent adult into society. The process is not without its birth pangs. If we follow the analogy we will accept that the birth is inevitable and the adolescent must break from the family, and that he should add his own activity, as does the foetus, to achieving the birth. Adolescence is only a very short section of a lifespan, yet it draws more attention and raises more heat than any other time of life. Many adults see adolescence as an awkward period to be lived through and got over as rapidly as possible, but it has a number of very important functions.[2]

As a period of transition it may bring an unique freedom from a number of established social restraints. As a child, the individual is firmly held within the structure and standards of his family.

---

[1] See pages 145–8 for training, supervision and support.
[2] Mays, J. B. (1965) *The Young Pretenders*. London: Michael Joseph.

As he becomes an adult and sets up home and nurtures a family of his own, he will again be surrounded by a similar settled situation with its own controls. For a few years he is foot-loose, neither child nor adult, and often without a settled stake in the fortunes of the community. It is as a result of this freedom from restraints and commitment that the adolescent and young adult has a special function to perform in questioning the manner of life and mores of his community. This is particularly important in more complex societies and during periods of rapid technological change, especially since social institutions tend to lag behind technological change. Adolescents may reject the accepted premises as a basis for their thinking and discussion. That all discussion should proceed from broadly agreed premises is part of what is meant by being 'within the establishment', and many adolescents are foot-loose in this respect also.

However uncomfortable or inconvenient, the contribution that can be made by its young people is indispensable to a changing society. But they will not be able to make this contribution unless they are held in a dialogue with the adult community, although this should not be held so closely as to neutralise their capacity to be different and to disturb.[1] In his 1970 Reith lectures, 'Change and Industrial Society', Dr D. A. Schon was in no doubt that the youth movement had caused some fundamental changes in American society.[2]

The adult population is at present finding it difficult to offer wise words of guidance to a new generation who will be coping with a very different and still rapidly changing world. New technologies are having a fundamental impact on accepted modes of life. There has been a revolution in communication, an invasion of the family living space by television, and there has been a spectacular increase in mobility of every kind. In the past, the families who moved their domicile in order to follow their work were mainly middle class; with the decline of traditional industries many more working-class families are joining this movement. The family car and other personal transport has

[1] Musgrove, F. (1964) *Youth and the Social Order*. London: Routledge and Kegan Paul.
[2] Later published in an enlarged version: Schon, D. A. (1971) *Beyond the Stable State*. London: M. Temple Smith. See also Hechinger, G. and F. M. (1964) *Teenage Tyranny*. London: Duckworth.

greatly increased individual mobility, and young people have been in the van of this development. Many young people have access to either car or motor cycle, with the result that within a few minutes drive they can be away from the eyes of people who know them, and from what were the traditional controls of the closer community. This has had the effect of making urban life even more impersonal.

Changing technologies have invaded the realm of human relationships in an even more direct way. More certain methods of birth control and more effective treatment of venereal diseases are having their effect on sexual relationships, and are likely to touch most dramatically our young people who are least held by established conventions. And any attack on the established controls of sex and procreation is likely to cause reverberations throughout the field of human relationships. Even the legislator is caught up in the tide, in legalising abortion. New moral issues will be awaiting the younger generation, for increased mobility and freedom from outside constraints bring not only new opportunities but also new responsibilities for personal judgement and choice. Morality is becoming less a matter of community control and precept, and much more one of personal decision, and in this sense life is becoming more democratic.[1] There is reason to doubt whether our educational system is offering young people enough help in their preparation of this kind of democratic living.

The greater mobility and the more impersonal nature of society has other implications. In a more static society the individual's social containment is almost structured for him within an immediate neighbourhood, but in a mobile society, with its looser structure and freer choice of relationships, the individual is not presented with the opportunity—almost the necessity—for stable relationships with anything like the same certainty. In our research we have found that many young people, who as children were happily settled in a network of relationships in their immediate neighbourhood, have been at a loss when their family has moved home or their position has become unsettled in some other way. It seems that they had the ability to respond to the peers whom they could scarcely avoid in a settled situation, but lacked the capacity to make the running in new circumstances. It appears from this that the new mobility may call for new

[1] Hemming, J. (1969) *Individual Morality.* London: Nelson.

social skills which present the school with new objectives for social education.

There is another kind of mobility that calls for similar social skills: I refer to the personal change in individual people looking to one another for some kind of close relationship. In a slowly moving society it is likely that the partners in, say, a marriage would change only slowly and would do so together. The case with a married couple who go in different directions to follow their own careers may be quite different. Both partners may be meeting a range of important but different experiences that have a considerable influence on their personal feelings, attitudes and behaviour. These experiences may be private rather than common, and can easily cause the partners to be changing in different directions. The success of the marriage will depend upon each accommodating to the other's change, but this is not likely to happen unless there is easy communication between them at a personal level. Many people find intimate conversation difficult, and this too seems to be a social skill of growing importance as the freedom, pace and mobility of life increases.

There is a tendency for young people to declare their independence of their homes earlier, and to join the adult community later, partly as a result of certain social forces, but also from their own volition. During this intermediate period they tend to be very dependent for support upon their peers, and their peer groups are likely to share a wide young people's sub-culture. Although in this they may keep their distance from the established community, they are certainly not left to their own devices: they are subject to the persuasive forces of commercial interest.[1]

Feelings about authority

Within this social setting many adolescents face a personal crisis of identity in a number of ways.[2] Their relationships to authority

[1] Abrams, M. (1961) *Teenage Consumer Spending*. London: London Press Exchange.
Packard, V. (1957) *The Hidden Persuaders*. London: Longmans.
[2] For a sympathetic discussion of adolescence, see Odlum, Doris (1961) *Journey through Adolescence*. Harmondsworth: Penguin Books.
For a series of papers leading into a more serious study of adolescence, see University College of Swansea, Faculty of Education (1966) *The Psychology of Adolescence*.

figures and their own future role in this respect looms large with many of them, and only those who have had the opportunity to explore their own feelings towards authority are likely to appreciate the full force of these feelings.[1] They have their roots in the young child's relationships with his parents, and when we watch a baby with its parents it is possible to see that his parents must seem to him almost omnipotent in their strength and power. The way in which parents exercise their authority is likely to have long-term effects, and recent research has demonstrated the influence of the parent's methods of communication and control on the general behaviour and expectancies of the child.[2] Some parents, more often of the middle class, reason with their children when trying to influence their behaviour, whereas other parents, more often of the working class, proceed by unexplained orders and precepts.

Many young people are in obvious difficulty in their attitudes to people in authority, and project their confusion on to the authority figure as if he were the cause of their anger. There is little doubt that some people do exercise their authority with incredible ineptitude, and the prevailing climate is inducing less acceptance of authoritarian behaviour, but basically the youngster expresses, in his reaction to the person in authority, his own feelings. This can be seen clearly when two youngsters react quite differently to the same authority situation.

With many adolescents their feelings about authority are bound up also with their attempts to declare their independence of their homes. And although they may rebel against authority, it is quite likely that their past experience will have sown in them an expectancy that deference should be paid to them when they become the person in authority. Some young people, particularly some working-class youngsters, may be making a very rapid transition from submissiveness or rebelliousness towards authority in the authoritarian family situation of their childhood to assuming a similar posture of authority in the family situation that they are about to create.

[1] Bazalgette, J. L. (1971) *Freedom, Authority and the Young Adult.* London: Pitman.
[2] Swift, D. F. (ed.) (1970) *Basic Readings in the Sociology of Education.* London: Routledge and Kegan Paul. (Chapter 14.)
Bernstein, B. B. (1965) 'A Socio-linguistic Approach to Social Learning'. In *Penguin Survey of the Social Sciences.* Harmondsworth: Penguin Books.

Vocational identity

For most young people, the transition from school to work is a period of some stress and uncertainty, though they may also find the experience of starting work both enjoyable and exciting. It depends upon how clear-sighted they are about what they want to do, or how well prepared for their chosen occupation, and, even more important, whether there is a suitable range of jobs available. Individual youngsters may be caught up in a period of uneasiness, very uncertain about their vocational role and sometimes suffering because of quite unrealistic expectations.[1] And since society at large tends to accord status on the basis of occupation, this is of vital importance to the way a young person wishes to see himself in the future.

'Vocational role' would seem a euphemistic way of describing the lot of many young people, for the choice of occupation is extremely limited in some districts, and those giving 'vocational guidance' have a thankless task. All kinds of irrelevant considerations enter the choice, such as a determination to work with friends, or a parent's preconception of what is a socially acceptable job. For some of the less able youngsters, the job that is available to them is a further confirmation of their lack of social worth, and it does not help that some of them seem to be actively seeking that confirmation. There are a few, particularly amongst the boys, who find it very difficult to settle down to a steady job at all. This is often caused by the very same kind of impediments, particularly a lack of effort, persistence and adaptability, that disturb them in other facets of life. Troubles rarely come singly.

When the first flush of excitement at earning money of their own has passed, the job palls for many youngsters; a period of uneasiness may follow and some may try their hands at several jobs before they settle down. Some are unsettled not so much by the nature of the work as by the behaviour of the adult workers they meet. Many girls especially have confessed to having been shocked by their contact with older married women: some of our respected 'mums' can be extraordinarily uncouth and almost vicious when with other women in an industrial setting. All too little attention has been given to the support of young people as

[1] Carter, M. P. (1966) *Into Work*. Harmondsworth: Penguin Books.

B

they venture into work. The contact between the youth worker and the youth employment service is at best patchy, and often non-existent, and the kind of interest shown by the youth worker is often typified by such statements as 'I got him a job at . . .' A much greater awareness is required of the pressures being faced by an individual young person in settling into that aspect of life which is going to do so much to determine his total social status and, in the fullness of time, that of his wife and family as well. And with that awareness should go appropriate enquiry and action, especially in terms of support, not only on the part of the educationist but also in industry. Much more attention should be given to pastoral functions in industry, especially for the semi-skilled and unskilled young worker.

Sexual and gender roles

The process of sexual maturation during adolescence, and the arousal of sexual interest and even disturbance that accompanies it, is a familiar subject.[1] Mating behaviour and the dealings between the sexes have been far less studied and described. Strong peer group control sometimes enters into mating, and individual young people may be far from free to approach members of the opposite sex in their individual manner. Mating displays and controls are sometimes so strong that it can only be assumed that the whole process is very highly charged for many youngsters. For example, a group of fifteen-year-old girls in a club had a routine of clowning and display that had the obvious purpose of attracting the attention of the boys around them. Yet when one of their number showed signs of making more personal contact with a particular boy, they would clutch her back into their circle and neutralise the developing relationship.[2]

In other peer sub-cultures, groups of boys have been known to have limited to a superficial level the relationship that any one of their number may establish with a particular girl. The controls of this kind of group may decree that sexual relationships should be only a casual series of events. In some cases the control can

[1] Schofield, M. (1965) *The Sexual Behaviour of Young People.* London: Longmans.
[2] Speed, B. (1968) Unpublished manuscript. University College of Swansea, Faculty of Education Library.

appear almost vicious, with members of the group feeling it incumbent on them to use girls sexually, and to boast of their exploits, whatever the reality may be.[1] In a Scout-Guide group a series of taboos had grown up that caused sexual relationships within the group to be avoided as if they were a mild form of incest.[2] Studies of mating behaviour give the impression that, in spite of the more open attitude of the community at large and the emancipation of young people, sex is still a tricky experience to handle.

There are often very few opportunities for boys and girls to gain experience of one another except through sexual and mating play. In many youth clubs there is a self-imposed segregation, and little within the structure of the organisation ensures that there will be opportunities for boys and girls to meet one another around neutral though personal topics. In many schools, too, opportunities are minimal; indeed the routine and often the seating does much to establish a taboo. It is not uncommon to see a boy or girl, brought into contact with the opposite sex as part of school life, ridiculed for it by his or her peers. Although coeducational schools make contact easier, merely bringing boys and girls together under one roof does not of itself provide suitable points of contact.

This is a matter that requires some attention. It is not helpful if boys and girls are almost forced, by the social controls around them, to begin a relationship through sexual exploration in some dark corner. Usually, the situation is not difficult to change. Some understanding of the forces at work is required, and a number of the techniques and strategies described later in this book could be employed. It is also not always realised, in this age of seeming enlightenment, that some young people are without the most elementary sexual knowledge.[3]

Peer roles and relationships

Older adolescence is a time of considerable mobility in friendship and of wider companionship; many young people may be under

[1] Jordan, J. (1970) Unpublished manuscript. University College of Swansea, Faculty of Education Library.

[2] Button, L. (1969) *The Seniors*. Swansea: University College of Swansea, Department of Education.

[3] Hacker, Rose (1966) *Telling the Teenagers*. London: Andre Deutsch.

some stress on this account, and some may even experience real unhappiness. The movement from school to work, or to establishments of further education, sometimes taking individual young people to new districts, may break contacts that have been settled for as long as ten years and throw individuals into a completely new circle of contacts. Access to a motor cycle or family car, desirable though this may seem, may hasten the end of settled groups. Mating adds to the process, and can cause a group to break up piecemeal, which can be especially painful for those left behind.

I am not wishing to suggest that these changes are harmful or unfortunate, or that it would contribute more to the welfare of young people if they were to retain their old contacts. Inevitable changes may threaten the social security of one person, but offer opportunities for new experiences and richer relationships to another. In some older working-class districts the neighbourhood structure is so close that friendship groups do survive the changes, and it might be more helpful to some of the youngsters concerned if the controls of their immediate groups were relaxed somewhat. In more loosely structured communities, as, for example, on some new housing estates, the changes may have a considerable effect on the patterns of relationships. In all this the youngsters of more limited social capacity may suffer periods of considerable malaise. The basis for friendship groups may change from the inescapable meeting at school and on the street corner to more deliberately planned meetings. The change tends to accentuate the difficulties of those with less social skill.

Adolescence as a time of emphasis

The difficult behaviour of young people in adolescence is often attributed to their being adolescent. In most cases it will be true that the stresses of adolescence will highlight certain aspects of their behaviour, but it cannot be emphasised too strongly that what they are portraying by their exaggerated behaviour may be a settled part of their long-term personalities. During adolescence the manifestation of their personalities may be etched rather more deeply than at other stages of life, but we do them no service by regarding their troubles as a function of adolescence that is to be got over as soon as possible. It is just as likely that they will be suffering similar stresses of personality in middle age.

Adolescence may be a moment when we can do more than at most other times in life to help people in their development, and the state of disturbance and flux should be seen as an opportunity rather than as a nuisance. Young people are also experiencing a brief freedom from some of the restraints that are to be with them at every other stage of life; and this, too, may be helpful in allowing change to take place. Might we not even describe adolescence as a 'melting pot' period of life, with unique opportunities for personal development? Since most of the help needed is in terms of the individual's responses to other people, the peer structure may provide both opportunities for practice in this, and support for experience and experiment in relationships outside the group.

The individual and the people who surround him

For individual development to take place there must be some personal freedom as well as support from others, but personal freedom is more than an absence of external restraint: the individual must also be free of internal compulsions or inadequacies.

As soon as we scratch beneath the surface we shall find, in most situations, people who are living rather less fully than they would like because of the limitations within their own personalities and of the lack of social skills.

Tiny was very large. He had no close friends. His approach to his peers was always very awkward and earned him repeated rejection, though he pressed himself on others continually. He confessed that he had been hurt as a boy by repeated references to how fat he was.

Sylvia was extremely shy to the point of being physically nauseated by having to meet new people. She had no close friends, and her life shuttled between a repetitive job and household chores. Conditions at home were difficult.

Jake was singled out by his rather shapeless figure and rubbery face. He served as a scapegoat wherever he went, and clearly provoked his peers into bullying him.

Janet was the self-appointed clown of her group. She would sabotage any serious conversation, and was seen by the staff at school as the leader of mischief. She seemed to relish the prominence—even the punishment—that her behaviour brought to her.

Josh was a particularly helpful boy to the adult leader of his youth group, and was the undisputed leader amongst his peers, a role that was obviously characteristic of him. In private conversation he confessed to a longing for close friends and to being lonely sometimes.

Beattie tried over-hard to please, and was quite unaware of the reaction of her peers to her inappropriate efforts to make herself acceptable.

But none of these people is an island; they are surrounded by others, particularly by their peers, who are adding their own reinforcement to the victim's personal inadequacies.

Tom had been a very violent boy at school and was the accepted leader of a small, violent gang. He had reached a stage when he would dearly have liked to escape this position, but whenever he was together with the members of that gang he found himself firmly in the same role.

Susan said that she had never dared to do anything different, interesting or adventurous, and she would really like to try. But when she was in the club with her friends, she firmly sat with them, their backs against the wall in a state of dynamic inactivity—'dynamic' inactivity because any attempt to change the situation was quickly neutralised.

Graham had earned the reputation for leading the mischief in school by his clowning. He confessed that he would have liked to take his school work more seriously, but never a lesson went by without his being reminded of his reputation either by his peers, or by a member of staff or both. And he was constantly pressed into his customary role.

Group roles and norms

In a settled social situation the individual's customary form of behaviour will arise from the interplay of his own personality and the controls operating in the group. This is rarely a deliberate process. Certain behaviour is repeated, becomes the normal and expected thing, and other members of the group adjust themselves to that expected behaviour. Members of the group are then not prepared or allowed to depart from the customary behaviour.

Beyond the accepted expectancies about the behaviour of individual people there will be more generalised forms of behaviour expected of the group as a whole. These expectancies are usually called group norms.[1] They may be seen in a more obvious and overt form in manners of dress and speech and in the routine of the group, but the norms of a group may also operate with great subtlety.

> Truancy in the lower ability forms seemed quite out of control. It was a matter of pride that no one should be at school for more than three days in any one week, and there was an elaborate myth current about the routine of the 'boardman'—the school attendance officer—and how to avoid attracting his attention.
> The boys of this village group seemed to be merely using the girls. None of them was expected by the group to form any lasting attachment to a girl, but he would be expected to extract some sexual reward for offering transport or escorting a girl for an evening. Whether or not he was successful in his designs, he was bound to report the success of the venture.

The sanctions that support these group norms may well be built into the normal life of the group, and some of them may be very sharp indeed.

> Sheila had stayed at home because the others had not called for her. She was very upset by what she saw as a response to something she had done or had not done.
> Although the routine of the group was repetitive and boring it had to be seen as a 'great time'. Anybody who missed an evening was told, when next seen by the group, that he had missed a 'really great night' though in fact it had been very like, and just as dull as, all the other evenings.

Personal uncertainty about our identity and place in life may make us particularly vulnerable, and social controls, especially those of peers, may bear very strongly on some adolescents.

[1] Klein, J. (1956) *The Study of Groups*. London: Routledge and Kegan Paul. (Chapter 6.)
Homans, G. C. (1951) *The Human Group*. London: Routledge and Kegan Paul. (See especially pages 118–28.) See also the section which follows, *Norms and Attitudes*, page 26.

Norms and attitudes

In considering group norms, special attention needs to be given to the level of acceptance of group norms amongst the members of the group. Although they may all conform equally, some may have their own reservations about what is happening. There is a difference between merely *complying* with group norms (and keeping our own counsel) and *accepting* them as valid and justifiable. As the strength of our commitment grows we may *identify* with what goes on (that is, accept it as our own), and there may be a further stage when we *internalise* a norm and respond unconsciously and spontaneously as if the norm had become part of us.

At this stage the internalised norm shades into our attitudes. An attitude is a predisposition to act in a certain way when faced by specific situations or people.[1] So many of our attitudes are caught from the people whose norms we share. Attitudes tend to be persistent and resistant to change. They are rarely held in isolation, but will be in interlocking systems of attitudes, which means that any change in one induces a ripple effect in others. Many of our attitudes are emotionally charged and are linked with our basic personality.

Attitudes and group norms may not coincide. Indeed there may be conflict between the individual's attitudes and the behaviour he accepts as the price of his membership of certain groups. To some extent the attitudes that we share with one group may set limits to what we may accept in another situation, but we may conform to the norms of a group in spite of our unspoken disagreement with norms that conflict with our established attitudes.

Helping through group work

Problems outlined on pages 23-5 arise largely through individual personalities, but the responses of the people around each individual have become so settled that he is no longer free to change even if he desires to do so. When an individual moves in several different circles he may behave differently in one situation from

[1] Jahoda, M. and Warren, N. (eds) (1969) *Attitudes*. Harmondsworth: Penguin Books.

another, but if some people are common to all those situations, his expected stereotype may firmly follow him. In any case, his role will probably have some basis in his own personality, and it is quite possible that he presents himself in a similar way wherever he goes. There is little point in trying to help someone in isolation if his difficulties are embedded also in the roles that he assumes in the groups to which he belongs, for in that case the individual and the people who surround him must change together.

Some work with young people may be approached most economically through case work or individual counselling, but some of their most basic problems concern their relationships, not least their difficulty in maintaining close and intimate relationships with peers. Many of those in greatest difficulty seem to be able to relate to the adult confidant or case worker, or even to those in authority. If new social skills must be learnt, or old habits modified, a group of people will be required as a laboratory for experience and experiment.

In this account there has been an emphasis on adolescents who have problems, and there is a danger of losing sight of the unrealised potential in so many 'normal' adolescents—or in all of us, for that matter. The same arguments apply: in so far as development concerns their relationships with other people, it can be approached most effectively by providing opportunities for experience and experiment in the company of other people. Group work means the deliberate use of group situations for this purpose.

The actual work may be approached in a number of different settings, and this book deals both with work with small groups in face-to-face situations, and with the kind of work that can be carried on in larger groups or institutions.

CHAPTER THREE

Making contact

In perspective

If we have an ambition to help young people to grow, to increase in their social effectiveness, possibly to achieve greater social adjustment, and to develop a sensitivity to and concern for others, then we are necessarily trying to involve them in a modification of their long-term behaviour. Behaviour, in turn, is bound up with their attitudes and ultimately with their basic personality. This is indeed a formidable undertaking.

The opportunities for developmental group work are to be found wherever groups of young people are gathered together; in Britain the greatest immediate potential is within schools and youth organisations, and in street and neighbourhood work. In many of these situations the contact will be entirely voluntary on the part of the youngster. If it is in a youth club, the length of contact with a particular group of young people may not be more than a few months or even weeks, and in street work the contact may be tenuous and brief. Anything we do must also compete with young people's other interests, and a sudden whim may take them beyond our reach. Even in school the work has to be fitted into a very full timetable, and the amount of time available to the worker and the group may be strictly limited.

We must therefore look for ways of accelerating our work if we are to achieve anything real in the time available. There has been a tendency for some group workers to approach their task so cautiously that their clients have left them before the work has had any real effect; indeed, there have been accounts of group workers spending many weeks in certain situations without making any real contact with possible clients.[1] This kind of leisure is not for us; a certain urgency must characterise our making contact as it does the rest of our work.

Reconnaissance

When preparing this chapter I considered the advisability of discussing reconnaissance at this point or at the end, for there is always a danger that what begins as necessary reconnaissance may be prolonged into procrastination, and serve as a pretext for not getting on with one of the many urgent jobs that we have identified. In any case the real needs of individuals, of groups, and even of neighbourhoods, will not reveal themselves to the observer from outside; quite soon reconnaissance shades into diagnosis, and once diagnosis has begun we are already at work. So may I make a plea that we do not spend very much time skirting around the situations that need our attention.

An outside assessment is usually quite quickly made, especially if other local workers can suggest possible starting points to us. For example, the worker-in-charge of a youth club can usually point to areas of need which help to focus the attention of the worker who is new to the situation, and the staff of most schools are very well aware of the trouble spots though they may not be so aware of social inadequacy. It is true that what is obvious to the observer may be a symptom of something much deeper, but the worker is not likely to discover this until in the course of his work his diagnosis has penetrated well below the surface.

Reconnaissance offers opportunities for influence that should not be neglected; it should be regarded as an integral part of the on-going work with the people we are hoping to serve. Just as I shall be suggesting that our diagnosis should be an experience that we share with the groups with whom we work, so we may view our reconnaissance as a means of involving other people in a study of their own situation and problems. This could be especially appropriate if we were, for example, hoping to involve the wider community in helping the young people in their midst. Reconnaissance may thus be approached through shared

[1] Mary Morse described such a cautious approach in *The Unattached*, e.g. pages 86 and 107. (Morse, M. (1965) *The Unattached*. Harmondsworth: Penguin Books.)

enquiries, or through action research as described later in this book.[1]

A word of caution: be careful not to stir movement in too many directions at once. The ramifications of your work will increase rapidly enough as you develop it, and you will be anxious not to spread yourself so thinly as to prevent your having any real impact.

Observing small groups

How sharp are our powers of observation, how objective are we, and do we see actually what happens and not what we think should happen? Effective observation is a vital tool of our trade, not just at the point of making contact but even more as we become involved in the work. It must be part of our deliberate policy to train ourselves in observation, and although I should like to cover this topic at this stage of my treatment, I do not wish by doing so to suggest that we must or can accomplish our own training in observation before we start serious work. Certain things we shall only see as we become more deeply involved in our work.

In practising observation it is quite unnecessary to await some special occasion: our laboratory is all around us, wherever people are to be found, and we can take our practice in our stride. Choose something uncomplicated, and at first attempt watch intently for only a few minutes. As soon afterwards as possible set down an account of what you saw in the greatest possible detail, though at the same time make your notes as economical as possible. Economy is at the core of good recording. The opportunities are legion: the meal-table at home, the bus queue, in the café, at the station, in the train, or at one of those interminable committee meetings you have to attend. Repeat the exercise a number of times until it becomes a habit to notice what is going on around you. Here is an example of a simple piece of reported observation. This, of course, is written up in prose form to suit its inclusion here, but it may be quite sufficient to record it in note form.

It was Friday evening in late Autumn, in a youth club meeting in a special building attached to a school. Three girls sat on a

[1] Page 85.

low platform with their legs dangling. The platform was in a small hall in which there were approximately fifty youngsters, of whom six or seven pairs, mainly girls, were dancing. The lights were low, and records were being relayed by an amplifier played at a level that made communication difficult but not impossible. The girls were on the side of the platform, facing the side wall. They were all aged about fourteen to fifteen.

Girl one, nearest to the back of the platform, was dressed in jeans and a dark jersey. She was of medium build, plain of feature, with hair that just fell around her head in no special way. She sat motionless except for her steady chewing. She did not seem to be following any movement with her eyes, which seemed to be looking vacantly in front of her.

Sitting next to her, but with a small gap between them, was girl two, who was slim, mini-skirted and in bright colours. Her features were neat, and her face was mobile in its expressiveness, her fair hair gathered into a pony tail. Girl three was sitting close to girl two. She was well built and shapely, wearing a mini-skirt and tightly fitting cardigan. Her features were round, and there was a softness in her face as she half smiled in listening to her companion. Her hair was black and thick, and fell to her shoulders. The only jewellery worn by any of the girls was a brightly coloured ring worn on the right hand of girl two.

Girl two was chatting with girl three, easily and rapidly, and supporting her words with movements of her head and neat hand gestures. She looked intently at girl three as she spoke. Girl three inclined her head as if to hear her neighbour clearly, looked up at her from time to time, but looked mainly at her left foot which she moved up and down slowly as she listened. Occasionally she responded in speech, which she signalled by lifting her head slightly and looking at her neighbour, at which her neighbour immediately stopped speaking and listened to what was usually only a few words.

Suddenly a fourth girl darted to them, and with her elbow on the knee of girl three engaged the attention of them both in what she had to say. As suddenly as she had arrived she broke off her conversation in order to jerk at the sleeve of a boy who was passing, but resumed what she had to say when the boy shrugged her off. As the two girls began to respond to her she ran away, crossed the hall, and disappeared from view. The two girls resumed their conversation exactly as before they were disturbed.

In the meantime girl one had slipped off the platform, and, still chewing and looking straight in front of her, leaned with her back and one elbow on the platform. She paid no visible attention to the fourth girl, but after a few minutes lifted herself back on to the platform and continued to chew. A minute or so later she again slipped off the platform and crossed in front of the other two girls. As she did so she spoke a few words to them, but without looking directly at them, to which they responded by lifting their heads and looking towards her face. She continued to look straight in front of her as she crossed the hall.

When you have recorded your own observation, try to find someone to whom you can report what you saw. Make sure that you observe not only the broad sweeps of behaviour but also the more subtle events that may be indicative of what is below the surface. Construct for yourself a check list and make sure that you can answer a number of essential questions such as:

(a) Who were the people involved? (Note sex, age, signs of marital status, e.g. engagement or wedding rings; general build, movement and mannerisms; style of dress and ornamentation; facial expression as well as features: our faces may not only portray our feelings, but may also condition other people's initial response to us, and even our feelings towards ourselves.)

(b) Who took the initiative and who responded? Did the exchanges flow or were they halting and spasmodic?

(c) Were there signs—gestures, smiles, frowns, non-committal grimaces—that might indicate the kind of feelings the people had for one another? (These would be only *signs*; much more detailed enquiry will be required before we talk of *evidence*.)

(d) Were there indications of sub-grouping? What were the seating arrangements or other physical proximity? What was the overall pattern of exchanges or interaction? (You could actually sketch a few moments of this as in Figure 1, opposite.) Do not forget that interaction is not only in terms of speech: there are many kinds of non-verbal communication.

(e) How were any arrivals and departures dealt with by the group?

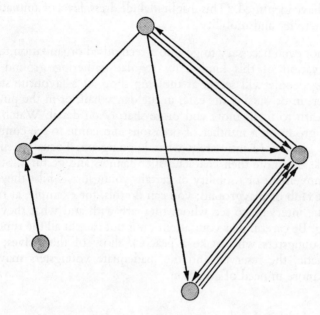

Figure 1 Interaction—a diagrammatic representation of a few minutes' exchanges between the members of a small group

Sub-structures within larger groups

I have just described what I would call *ad hoc* observation: a passage of activity in a small group that we may observe on only a single occasion. We shall need to extend this into longer and more systematic observation of groups meeting over a period. This you can practise by attaching yourself to some larger group that meets regularly, such as a youth club, and observing:

(a) the movement within the larger group;
(b) any collection of people that seems to occupy the same space from time to time;
(c) the interaction taking place within this collection of people;
(d) what happens if any of those people move away—where they go, how the remaining people respond, if they return, how they are received by those who have remained together;

(e)   any signs that would indicate that the collection of people you are watching is in fact a sub-group of a larger gathering;

(f)   any differences in behaviour between sub-groups that you have identified. (This might include dress, level of animation, activity and mobility.)

It is not even necessary to go into a recognised organisation to do observation of this kind. Any regular gathering ground for young people will serve: at the chip shop, at a favourite street corner, in or outside the café, in the dance hall, or in the pub.

Learn to focus more and more sharply on detail. Watch the same group on a number of occasions and come to see cumulatively and more intimately what is going on. Focus on single people, and note their characteristic manners and gestures. Study the movement or mobility of certain youngsters whilst they are in the club or playground; you can do this, for example, at two-minute intervals, to see whom they are with and what they are doing. Be careful that your attention is not caught all the time by the youngsters who make a peacock show of themselves; the apathetic, the reserved and the inadequate youngsters may be even more in need of attention.

Watching for signals

What is said is not necessarily the most potent part of the message; we convey a good deal by the tone in which we say things. For example, see in how many ways in which you can say, 'Do you think so, Joe?' to convey different messages. Can you by a different tone convey: straight enquiry, doubt, apprehension, ridicule, sympathy with Joe's position? This is happening all around us, and sometimes we convey the second message contained in the tone of speech quite unintentionally, but the group worker will need to be conscious of what is going on at the same time as he responds to it.

We convey a good deal also through our facial expressions. Watch a single person closely for a few minutes at a time. Start with eye contact—where does he look when addressing his companions; what messages does he convey through his eyes? Eye contact is a very powerful medium for communication, and the group worker in particular will need to be aware of the way he uses eye contact, especially when encouraging group discussion. In teaching or lecturing the use of the eyes is of great importance, and can make the difference between involving all one's audience or encouraging minds to wander. And just as we can engage people with our eyes, so we may withdraw from situations or deflect conversations by avoiding eye contact.[1]

We should be conscious of facial movement, and practise noticing every flicker: the mouth, the brows, eyelids and the general poise of the head are all indicators of thoughts passing through the person. At times a mere flicker may be the only signal offered to the worker that someone is ready for what may prove to be a very formative exchange in the development of that particular youngster. Gestures and movement are similar bearers of messages. Hands may be especially expressive, but we need also to notice more general body movement, including agitation or repose, briskness or sluggishness, and whether the movement is integrated or disjointed. The worker's effectiveness will depend on his skill in detecting the emotional undertone of what is taking place—the message within the message.

Observation must form part of the continuing practice of the group worker.

Choice of group

It is quite likely that we shall not really know whether we have chosen the right group until we have made some progress in our work with it. If we have attached ourselves to what seems to be a natural friendship or associate group, we may not realise until we have come to know the members well, or have conducted a sociometric study, that one or two of the most influential members of the natural circle are not with the group when members meet us.

We shall also need to consider whether we should work with an already existing associate or friendship group, or whether a group might be brought together on some other basis. We may take as our point of departure several young people who seem in obvious need of help; we shall then need to consider whether they are members of a natural associate group, and whether, in

[1] Argyle, M. (1967) *The Psychology of Interpersonal Behaviour*. Harmondsworth: Penguin Books. (Especially Chapters 2, 3, 5, 6.)
Button, L. (1971) *Discovery and Experience*. London: Oxford University Press. (Page 152.)

this case, the rest of the group would welcome the group worker, and benefit too from the experience. The youngsters may already be involved in an activity or task group, but before we approach them through this avenue we shall need to ask ourselves whether the task situation would be helpful or an impediment to the work. The preoccupation with a task can at times seriously impede the development of more personal and intimate conversation within the group.[1]

How are we to reach young people who are not attached to any small group or even to another person? An attempt to attach them to an already existing friendship group involves automatic difficulties, for not only may a friendship group tend towards exclusiveness, but we are also inviting the youngster, who may find relationships difficult, to make what may be the trickiest move of all. It is much easier to attach him to an activity, or task, or functional group, but this, too, faces us with the danger that concentration on a task may impede the more personal exchanges, and our whole purpose may be defeated.

It is possible to think in terms of a group brought together deliberately and admittedly for the purpose of group work, and to gather into this a number of people who would both benefit from it and agree to take part. But a group of this kind may have the disadvantage of not being an organic group which continues to support the individual in normal situations outside group meetings. The resolution of these dilemmas may reside in the manner in which the worker approaches his task, and in particular in his style of leadership.[2] Even a natural friendship group can see itself as a different group when it is with the worker, and may therefore make way for the person who is normally an outsider but who will be accepted by the group in this special context.

Workers are often faced with the problem of whether or not new members should be admitted to the group after they have started their experience with him, especially when he is working in an informal setting and encouraging the self-determination of the young people concerned. When members of a group have reached considerable intimacy in their discussions, it could easily be destructive for them to receive a new member who has not

[1] Foulks, S. H. and Anthony, E. J. (1965) *Group Psychotherapy*. Harmondsworth: Penguin Books. (Pages 33–7.)
[2] See page 39.

had the experience that led up to this situation. In practice it does not always work out like that: quite often a newcomer falls immediately into the general tone of the exchanges. Much will depend upon the preparation for the entry of the new person, and sometimes an invitation to a new member is issued by the group out of concern for that person.

I shall be returning later to the question of the size of the group,[1] and the circumstances that favour working with a natural friendship group or a contrived group will become clearer as the discussion of the work proceeds.

A direct approach

Having come to some provisional decision about the group of people with whom we wish to work, how do we make contact with them? It is at this point that there may be so much difference in the speed of work. I was brought up in the school that preached great caution at this point, lest we alienate the young people with whom we wish to work: 'Don't ask questions, just stick around', seemed to be the philosophy. But as we developed our research, which necessitated an immediate contact with young people at a fairly intimate level, we began to question our previous caution. The contact that we made as researchers was usually warm and immediate, and as we developed studies that necessitated more sustained contact with young people, we found that we were doing more effective 'group work' as researchers than we were as group workers. As result of this we changed our approach, and even used similar forms of enquiry as a basis for our initial point of contact and for the ensuing work.

To the reader who is dubious about the possibility, the effectiveness, or about the ethics of this kind of direct approach, I can only suggest that he tries it for himself. Consider the basic minimum information required in order to work intelligently with young people, and incorporate this into a form of enquiry. The questions will be factual and objective, but can be so framed that they edge on to areas of concern and intimacy so that the youngster may take the conversation further if he wishes. In conducting interviews as part of group work, we use forms of enquiry as prompts for a flowing conversation rather than a

[1] See page 105.

question and answer session, and we would readily depart from a preconceived order of topics if the spontaneous conversation with the youngster led us to do so.[1]

If you are going to try this for yourself, consider carefully your approach, and if possible get someone to help you role-play how you will make your first contact with a youngster and conduct the interview. Learn to focus on the youngster: if he occupies your full attention your own anxieties and hang-ups will fall away. When you meet the youngster, let yourself into the situation gracefully but don't beat about the bush. We find that most young people prefer a direct and honest approach; prevarication and pretence only build barriers. Assure the person of the confidentiality of what he tells you, and as you proceed make it easy for him not to answer anything that he would prefer to avoid.

Whether we are meeting a whole group or individual youngsters, we follow the practice of declaring our identity at the outset, and in particular we try to convey our personal interest in them. It is unlikely that they can foresee at this stage what the contact may lead to, but most are prepared to accept us on trust, or merely on the basis of our personal interest in them and the immediate conversation with us. Many groups of youngsters have responded to us as if they had been waiting for one of our breed to turn up!

In this way it is possible to move into deep and concerned conversation even at the first meeting; we have found that the long periods of 'going along with' young people, reported by a number of group workers, are quite unnecessary. Nor have we found it necessary to resort to such devices as establishing coffee bars in order to make contact with any specific groups of young people—if we have wanted to meet certain youngsters we have merely gone out to meet them. Naturally we see that they are always in the position to choose whether they wish to continue contact with us.

We have made a direct approach to all kinds of youngsters in many places in Britain and in several other countries. Occasionally we are rebuffed, but have learnt to see this as a point of

[1] For a discussion of the kinds of prompts that might be included in an initial form of enquiry, see pages 44–6. The use of forms of enquiry in training is discussed in Button, L. (1971) *Discovery and Experience*. London: Oxford University Press, including some examples in Appendix 2.

departure for a new approach; it is rare that contact cannot be made, and sometimes it is at a special level because of the initial rejection. We feared at first that this kind of approach would be rejected by the more difficult and anti-social youngsters, but they are often the easiest to contact in this way and respond with the most interest and vigour. In general, few youngsters fail to respond to the genuine interest in them expressed by the worker. Some have themselves brought together the group that has formed the basis for the work.

The worker's fear of rejection is often the greatest impediment to his effectiveness, and those training themselves to work in this direct manner may need the support of a supervisor or a group of colleagues. It is not that they should be saved the pain of being rejected, but they need to be helped to come to terms with their fears; it is often helpful for the worker to see that the rejection of him is as a functionary rather than as a person. And the day that the worker tells himself that it is his own timidity that is the main impediment to his progress is usually a turning point in his effectiveness.

It is important to see the first contacts as an early stage of an on-going diagnosis, which has the immediate effect of adding greater depth and meaning to the conversations.

The worker's leadership

The essence of group work is more in what transpires between the members of the group than in the relationship between the individual members and the group worker. Therefore, at the same time as making contact with the members of the group, the worker will be seeking some point of focus that will help the group to act together. We have called this focus the 'context' of the group: from the Latin root *contexere*—'to weave together'.

The context of a group, their activity, or the focus for their interaction, is at every stage a very important factor and not least at the beginning of the work. There will need to be a context that will not only hold the group together, but will do so with the worker within it. This is well illustrated by the natural friendship group. If the main context of the group is restricted to the expression of friendship for one another, then there is only the most precarious toe-hold for the worker, no matter how willing the group are to accept him.

This raises the whole question of what kind of leadership should be offered by the group worker. There is a tendency on the part of some group workers to want to deny that they are in a position of leadership at all; often they equate 'leadership' with strong direction. The exercise of leadership is a matter of some complexity, and includes the sharing of leadership with the members of the group. Presumably the group worker's purpose is to influence the group, and therefore he cannot be just one other member of the group.

I have already referred to the tendency of some group workers to 'go along with' their groups. This usually arises either from the worker's timidity or from his policy of keeping his initiative to the minimum. It also usually implies that the group continues to focus upon its existing context, with the inevitable result that the worker rather lamely trails along with the group without any real place in it, almost as a foreign body. If he is going to have real influence, his position will need to be considerably stronger than this, and such strength can only be achieved if the context accepted by the group makes a place for him. Workers have reported that it is all too easy to be drawn into sharing the boredom of an apathetic group. The worker in this position is really being drawn into the influence of the group's existing normative controls, with the result that he has the double job, first of breaking free from the controls that he has allowed to crystallise around him, before, second, he begins to help the group to move.

When a worker first joins a group, his intrusion is likely to disturb the existing certainty about what is to be expected. There may be a certain hiatus, a brief suspension of certain normative controls during which the group may be led towards new forms of behaviour. This moment of flexibility is an important part of the worker's capital, which may evaporate as the group rapidly evolves a new framework of expectancies or reverts to the old. It may be very much harder to win so much flexibility once the situation has been allowed to crystallise.

It is not always appreciated just how strong an influence is being exerted by existing normative controls. For example, a group may have a repetitive and boring routine, and their inactivity and apathy may be embedded in the firm expectations held of one another. To move a group of this kind to a different level of expectations may require fairly stirring leadership. At other times the controls may be part of a situation that surrounds the group. We have found this frequently when working in youth clubs. In some clubs the prevailing group norms may neutralise any attempts to encourage young people to engage in long-term activity and initiative, and it is sometimes necessary to encourage them temporarily to move out of this familiar situation in order to break through the rigid controls. In school situations where the general attitudes of the pupils have been unhelpful, we have found it necessary so to change the setting that the youngsters were momentarily disorientated, and the usual rigid controls were suspended. Once a new normative structure has been established, it seems possible for this to survive like an oasis within a larger establishment.

Inexperienced workers often suffer a good deal of anxiety and frustration in the early stages of their work with a group. When working in an entirely voluntary situation, such as in the street or in a youth club, the worker may not even be sure he will see his group again. Unless he can encourage them to involve themselves in a fairly compelling context, he may fail to get them to gel as a group that includes him, and may even lose contact with them altogether. Many workers find this a more difficult stage to work through than making the initial contact. Contrary to what is often thought, the worker is more likely to lose contact with young people through his indefinite leadership than by attempting to engage them in a fairly positive way.

I have so far written in general terms about the importance of the context without suggesting what the context might be. I shall be suggesting in Chapter 5 that it should lead to that kind of experience most economically addressed to the more urgent needs of the young people concerned, but at the outset it will be difficult to assess what this might be. It is helpful if the contexts can arise out of any strong feelings within the youngsters, and workers soon learn how to batten on to something that seems to stir the group. As we start to work we may feel grateful for anything that promises to bring the youngsters a useful experience and gives us time to fumble around for something with better long-term possibilities.

At times the worker may find that he is himself the only effective context, and that the group will continue mainly because of his interest in them, or their attachment to him. This may imply that the youngsters are expressing a dependence upon the worker, and it is not unusual, when a worker first comes to realise this, for him to draw abruptly back. There is a lot of confusion about this, as there is also about how strong a leadership should be offered. It is most important that events should be seen as part of a long-term programme. If a young person is ultimately to achieve self-reliance, he may need the worker's—and the group's—close support on the way.

If the worker approaches his task systematically, he will find that contexts which will grip the group present themselves automatically. This is particularly true of the early stages, as he begins serious diagnosis, but more of that in the next chapter.

Testing out

It is often found that at an early stage of their experience the youngsters will 'test out' the worker. This they may do by trying to shock him or her, or in some other way seeing just how far they can go. This may happen in particular with youngsters who are rebellious towards people in authority, and it may be a way of finding out whether the worker is just like all those other people in authority whom they dislike so much.

It is sometimes suggested that this is an inevitable stage of development, but in our experience the amount of testing out varies considerably from group to group, and more particularly from one worker to another, and seems to be influenced by the approach of the worker as much as by the nature of the group. It is often particularly strong when there is a lack of clarity in the group worker's position, especially when he offers indefinite or enigmatic leadership. Sometimes there is something of a T-group situation,[1] arising largely from inactive leadership, in which the group do not know what to make of the worker. In these circumstances it is hardly surprising that they test him out.

If the worker wishes to expose young people, as part of their experience, to situations that have uncertainty inherent in them, then this kind of leadership will certainly achieve it. But situations of this kind are sometimes created by workers who would eschew deliberate manipulation; indeed, it may arise from their efforts to avoid manipulation and from the resultant neutral position that they take up.

[1] See page 67.

CHAPTER FOUR

Social diagnosis

The need for clear and rapid diagnosis

It is possible to afford considerable help to young people merely by expressing a kindly interest in them and introducing them to a number of enlarging experiences; generations of men and women have brought the benefits of human warmth and kindness to young people in this unself-conscious way. Much the same can be said about the efforts of the many adults who have engaged young people in some activity that interested them personally. Nothing written in this book is intended to detract from the contribution that these people have made and are still making. In some ways they may have been more effective in their single-mindedness than more self-conscious workers, who may become inhibited by the possibility of their doing the wrong thing, or who have attempted to 'give young people opportunities for forming relationships' through a policy of studied inactivity.

No matter what part we play in service to young people, we are likely to work more effectively and economically if our objectives, and the paths to those objectives, are clear. Those objectives must surely reside in the needs of individual young people, in the way that they are held and supported by the people around them, and in the kind of contribution they make to others. Time and resources are limited, and it is therefore vital that we establish our objectives through a clear and rapid diagnosis.

Diagnosis is in part, but only in part, a gathering of information. Some of the picture, such as the behaviour of the youngster in certain situations of stress, we may only see by demonstrations over a period of time. We may be able to gather certain material through tests designed to illuminate areas of feeling and behaviour. And in some ways the youngster may be the best informant about himself through straightforward conversation, especially as he becomes more articulate. Being articulate is not merely a matter of having the language with which to describe events and feelings; there must also be insight that makes the identification of those feelings possible. Yet language is the instrument through which these feelings may be identified; thus insight and the acquisition of the necessary language must proceed together. We find that youngsters can grow in insight and become more articulate with striking rapidity, and are thus able to help us in our diagnosis.

The case for direct methods of making contact was argued in Chapter 3, and a similar case for a direct approach to social diagnosis can be made. Indeed the means of making contact and the initial diagnosis may coalesce. If a youngster agrees to tell us about himself, then the way is clear for important conversations, and besides being helpful to our work, the exchanges are likely to be fascinating and helpful to the youngster also. We have discovered during our research programmes that when we have had occasion to invite young people into a continuing dialogue with us over a period of time, many of them have benefited greatly from the experience.

About the individual

Clearly we need to know at the beginning of our contact something about the personal background of the youngsters we are working with, and to sense some of the more prominent attitudes they hold. What prompts would you establish for yourself in order to ensure that you were covering the necessary ground in a systematic way? Having asked this question of many groups of workers, I have found a recurring pattern emerging. Here are some of the main strands.

Identification We need to know name (including nickname?), sex, age, and address. There are often debates about whether we should ask for the address, especially when we are doing street work. In general we find that it is freely offered, and if we know our district it can at once tell us a great deal.

School The youngster's experience at school is important. The standards he has achieved may express both his natural ability and the kind of support (or lack of it) that he receives at home. It may also give hints about his personal willingness to learn, and the influence of his peers. We should really like to know something about his experience at school: his behaviour, his relationships with the staff, whether he enjoyed school, and how all this fits into his general outlook. It is sometimes suggested that questions about school focus on what may be a delicate topic, but this could be advanced as a good reason for including such questions rather than the reverse. We rarely experience any difficulty in leading young people into this kind of area, and they more often than not volunteer much more than we ask. Even the teacher who is doing some group work in his own school, with young people whom he normally teaches, seems to be able to take this kind of thing in his stride.

Work The youngster's work experiences are another important indicator. We need to know the level of work as well as occupation: for example, is it skilled or unskilled work, and is he an apprentice or a labourer? Any movement from job to job may lead to further conversation, and to a revelation of his general level of satisfaction or frustration in work, including his level of persistence or willingness to work.

Family background Family background may, for some, be an area of life that is highly charged emotionally. Questions about the occupation of the father, and whether the mother is following any occupation, usually reveal whether both parents are living at home, and sometimes a lot more besides. Questions about brothers and sisters by ages, with their school or work, and whether the family has moved, will add very considerably to the picture. A few factual and objective questions of this kind will open the way for the youngster who would like to use the worker as a confidant: young people with difficult home backgrounds are very often the keenest to do so.

Friends Do we enquire about friends at this early stage? We may intend later to enquire more deeply into friendships and other relationships, but a more general enquiry about friends as part of an early conversation often produces useful insights into the way the youngster lives his life. Sometimes he will volunteer immediate information about how he gets along with his peers. We find youngsters very ready to tell us whether they have a steady boy-friend or girl-friend.

General interests When we are considering our next moves, information about the youngster's interests and ambitions (or lack of them) may be crucial. This should include his affiliation to clubs and other organisations, and any further education he is following, including training commitments at work. We may wish to include here an enquiry about religious affiliation.

There is a lot more to an interview than getting information. When the interview has been completed the worker will need to stand back and tell himself what happened. How did the youngster behave? Were there indications of his attitude to parents, teachers, employers, peers, or in general to those in authority? What feelings about himself did he portray? By setting down a few notes about matters of this kind the worker will be able to bring the total personality of the interviewee into better focus.[1] In framing an enquiry, questions that skirt areas of strong feeling and attitudes can be particularly valuable. The worker who creates an unhurried atmosphere for his interview may be able to detect emotional undertones beneath what is being said, and to encourage the discussion of themes that the youngster feels are important to him. In this way the worker may learn much about the attitudes of the youngster to life and, for example, to authority.

We may be held back from prying out of a respect for the privacy of the youngster, but is it not rather a question of opening to young people opportunities to use the worker as a confidant should they wish to do so? By keeping the situation 'safe', by not approaching areas that may be charged emotionally, we may in practice be signalling that we are not prepared to share their anxieties and burdens. Many youngsters, who have obviously gained considerably from intimate conversations of this kind, have indicated to us that they would have liked a similar opportunity long before, but the youth workers or teachers with whom they were in contact had not led them into suitable conversations and thus opened the way for their confidences.[2]

[1] Garrett, A. (1948) *Interviewing, its Principles and Methods.* New York: Family Service Association of America (44 East 23rd Street, New York, N.Y. 10010).
[2] Button, L. (1967) *Some Experiments in Informal Group Work.* Swansea: Department of Education, University College of Swansea. (Page 10.)

Here we face what seems to be quite a basic principle of communication. It would seem necessary that the person who is senior in a partnership must open up the channels of communication before the junior partner will take the initiative. It is as if he must demonstrate that a particular area of conversation is legitimate. It is not enough to say that he is open to receive confidences: he must actually begin conversation that will have accustomed them both to exchanges in specific areas of intimacy. Examples of this can often be seen in family life. It is unusual for children in the family to open up new areas of intimate conversation—about sex, say—and the kinds of topics discussed will usually depend upon the conversation initiated by the parents. It also points to the uncertain position of, for example, youth workers who say that their club members know that they may bring any problems to them. Making ourselves available as a confidant is an active rather than a waiting game.

So far we have been dealing with overt events, conditions and behaviour, but many of the springs of behaviour are far less tangible. For example, has the youngster feelings of anxiety and guilt, and what are his feelings about his own social worth? What is his level of resilience to uncertainty, criticism and hostility? How would we describe his temperament? How socially timid or bold is he, what is his level of persistence, and how flexible and spontaneous is he? Is he sensitive to others and has he empathy and compassion? Later in this book I shall be suggesting tests and exercises that will help stimulate the investigation of personal behaviour and feeling. Much can be achieved through personal conversation and group discussion, so long as the worker approaches the occasion with a clear framework of enquiry, which may form a working agenda. This kind of exploration usually draws a ready response from young people, and can serve as a compelling context for the first few meetings of the group.

Any discussion that touches them personally is likely to grip young people. By using personal feeling as the focus for discussion, the worker may achieve a triple take: he gains vital insights for his own guidance; he engages young people in their own self-discovery; and he accustoms the group to open and intimate discussion in a supportive atmosphere. Topics like friendship—which leads so often also to loneliness—and intimate feelings of joys, hopes, anxieties, guilts and hostilities will readily serve this treble purpose.

Friendships and styles of relationships

In a sample survey we conducted to enquire into the problems that had been faced by some seventeen-year-olds who left school at the age of fifteen, we included a special group each of whom was said to have been a problem at school, and who would probably meet difficulties after having left school. We were surprised to find that this group of youngsters had faced comparatively fewer problems than the other young people interviewed, who had not been seen as problems at school. Although they may have presented problems to their school, most of them were making their way very nicely now that they were out in the world.

By far the greatest number of 'problems' were not those that would cause the youngster to be troublesome to other people: the greatest difficulties lay within the youngsters themselves. Nearly a quarter of those interviewed had a sense of inadequacy or malaise sufficiently serious to impair their quality of life. The greatest single difficulty mentioned was in making friends. This assessment is not based on the standards of middle-class observers, but on the testimony of the youngsters concerned. They made it clear that they were not content with their pattern of relationships, and in particular found friendship-making difficult. We have been increasingly impressed by the central and critical position that friendship-forming takes in the lives of young people. Not only does it seem to be the toughest relationship to strike up, but if young people are not adequately contained in their friendships, they may be in trouble in a number of other ways as well.

Their difficulty in forming friendships does not usually extend to every other kind of relationship: they may well be able to relate to adult confidants and sometimes have considerable social poise that makes them acceptable to adults and often to authority figures. Some youngsters substitute functional or task relationships for close friendships, which may range from the club chairman of great poise and ability[1] to the inarticulate leader of the violent gang. The little girl helping in the club coffee bar who remarked that it was 'safer behind the counter' was probably

[1] Button, L. (1969) *The Seniors*. Swansea: University College of Swansea, Department of Education. (Page 28.)

saying more than she knew. It is not uncommon to find this same combination of a lack of close friends and reliance on functional relationships in delinquent or near-delinquent groups of youngsters. It is as if they were gathered around the tasks of defence or offence, or of planning their 'jobs', as a substitute for real friendship. Could this difficulty in close relationships be one of the roots of true delinquency?

In the course of our research, young people have made it clear that they have friendships at various levels.[1] At the kernel are the intimate friends whom I shall call 'close friends'. Most youngsters have close friends; some have only one, but more have several; a few have six or more: they vary considerably in this respect. A very small number survive happily without any close friends at all, but most of those without close friends have told us that they regret their lack of friends, some of them very deeply.

Most youngsters have other friends whose company they seek and with whom they spend considerable time, but their relationship with these friends lacks the intimacy of the close friendship. I shall be calling this level of friendship 'other friends'. The difference between the two levels of friendship is in the trust and confiding nature of the close friendship, and most youngsters are clear about the distinction. The number of other friends is usually a little larger than that of close friends, but again this varies from one youngster to the next.

In addition to these friends, most youngsters have a number of companions who form part of their wider circle. Although they do not accept them as friends as described here, they gain comfort and pleasure from their company. They may not go around with them, but if they are in a club or dance hall, they may spend some time with them and then return to their friends. I shall be calling these more distant companions 'associates'. We may need to add the context in which they are met, because any single youngster may have several sets of associates as, for example, his associates at work, or in sport, or the crowd who 'hang out' at the same place as he and his friends, or even associates in crime.

The total pattern of friendship with which individual young people surround themselves may be very different from one to the

[1] Button, L. (1965) *Friendship Patterns of Older Adolescents.* Swansea: University College of Swansea, Department of Education.

next, and would seem to be characteristic of that person. What one sees at any particular moment is likely to be indicative of a long-term style of friendship that has its roots in the personality and social skills of that person. In studies of individual young people carried out over a period of time, it has been found that although the actual people named as friends may change, a very similar pattern of friendship has continued. If a particular friend should be lost as a result, for example, of a change in circumstances, it is as if the individual were left with a loose feeler which reaches out until it becomes attached to a new person. Or the status of someone already in his circle of companionship may change as, for example, from other friend to close friend. These characteristic styles of friendship are sometimes obvious for all to see. In common parlance we may refer to someone as a 'lone wolf', or be aware that 'he always has lots of friends about him', although we may be constrained to add in some cases, 'but his relationships always seem fairly superficial'. Helen Jennings has described the long-term manner in which the individual surrounds himself with friends as his 'emotional expansiveness'.[1]

It is possible to see 'friendship' as describing the qualities or actions of our friends, but it may be sounder to see it in terms of our own need for friends and our capacity to relate to them. It is almost as if we press the other person into a role that fits our own needs: the feeling for friendship is ours; the other person responds to us. The truth of this is etched clearly by the frequency with which people miscalculate the feelings of other people towards them. When one person names another as a friend he is really expressing his own feelings, and the person he names may not have reciprocal feelings towards him.

Friendship is often described in terms of reaching out to the other person, but we have come to see it even more as an opening up of ourselves to the other person, letting or inviting him into our intimate self. This may mean that anything within us that we do not wish other people to see, whether it is real or imaginary, may present an impediment to friendship-forming. I shall be returning to this in Chapter 7 when considering the help we may offer to young people who are in difficulties in making friendships.

The actual difficulties with friendship manifest themselves in a number of ways. I have already mentioned those young people

[1] Jennings, H. (1950) *Leadership and Isolation*. London: Longmans, Green.

who find refuge in relationships with adults, either as confidants or as people in authority, and a number relate to either older or younger people but never to their peers. Some rely almost entirely on functional or task relationships, but there are others who seek peer relationships yet, as a result of their own inept behaviour, are ignored or rejected. Youngsters of this kind are sometimes to be seen hovering around the fringe of one group after another. Some young people who earn persistent rejection appear to have converted this into the only kind of relationship that they can manage, and they would rather receive hostile attention, it would seem, than no attention at all.

If we are right in our assumption that a long-term style of relationships exists, this sets limits to the short-term help that can be offered to young people. For example, it is possible that our attempt to induce close friendship amongst a group with whom we are working might only succeed at the expense of certain friendships hitherto maintained outside the group. It will also disabuse us of any fond hopes that by merely bringing people together—giving them opportunities for making friends—we shall enable them to satisfy their need for friendship. Attempts to help them may require much more formative experience than that.

Friendship study

The way that the individual operates in a group gives us clues not only about his relationships but also about his personality. We shall want to know about the structure of the group as rapidly as possible, especially if we choose to work with an already existing group. We shall be interested in the whole range of relationships that exist in the group, the part that the group plays in the total lives of its members, the roles that are assumed by individual members, and the normative controls. Observation and intuition may lead us to a good deal of this, although we have learnt to be cautious about backing our general impressions, for more exact tests have often revealed that our observation has been at fault. For example, sociometric tests have frequently shown us to have been wrong in our judgement about the friendships existing in a number of groups with whom we were working.

One of the most useful ways of conducting a sociometric test for this purpose is through a friendship study. This will achieve several different objectives at the same time: it will reveal the

c

friendships within the group (or lack of them), and the total pattern of friendships surrounding each individual, which will include both the way he looks to the group for his friendships and the kind of social containment he enjoys outside the group. Most young people find the experience provided by the study valuable in itself.

Here are the descriptions of the levels of companionship that seem to draw ready response from young people:

Close friendship   Someone you like and probably meet frequently, whom you trust and rely on, to whom you would confidently tell secrets—and expect him to do the same to you.

Other friend   Someone you like and possibly meet frequently, whose company you seek, and who is more than an associate but not a close friend.

Associate   You may not go out of your way to meet this person, but if he happened to be about you would join up with him.

Acquaintance   Someone you would acknowledge upon meeting, but would not normally choose as a companion for a social occasion.

Although these descriptions are in our language and need to be interpreted in conversation with the young people concerned, they usually are soon expressing the spirit of the distinctions in their own way. For example, a close friend may be variously described as the person who 'really understands me', or 'my buddy', or 'someone I could borrow money from', or who would 'always back me up in a fight'.

In conducting a friendship study we normally restrict the categories to close friends and other friends. A brief conversation will distinguish these two levels, and we then ask the youngster to name his friends at each level. If we have a prepared form it is important that its layout—or our use of it—should not imply to the youngster that he is expected to produce a certain number of friends at each category: we need to assure him that people vary considerably in the number of friends they have.

Without much extra trouble it is possible to gather additional information of value to the worker, and increase the interest to the young person. For example, we might ask the following questions about each friendship.

How long have you been friends?

How did you first meet?

What do you do together?

Where does he/she live (giving district and distance)?

It is also helpful to enquire at this stage whether the youngster has a boy-friend or girl-friend, is going steady, is engaged, or married, to see how this enters the pattern of friendship that has been revealed. If there is the leisure, and we are wanting to make use of a study of this kind as an important experience for a group of young people, we can extend the enquiry into feelings for the other person:

What do you especially like about this friend?

Is there anything you dislike about him/her?

The conversation may be deepened further by considering whether any close friends have been lost in the recent past, and what caused the friendship to end.

We find it best to proceed through a conversation rather than straight question and answer, and this gives the youngster an opportunity, which most young people are eager to take, of exploring his friendships as the interview proceeds. Sensitive interviews of this kind, especially when the young person responds to the group worker as a confidant, can be of great value, but do depend on adequate time being available.

Where there is insufficient time for personal interviews, it is possible to complete a friendship study by working in a small group. In this case friendship, and the meaning of each category, will be the subject of group discussion in general terms, after which each youngster will complete the form, often raising queries and points of interest as he does so. This can give rise to a very happy and profitable occasion, and preserves the confidentiality of the study if this is what the group wishes to do. The least satisfactory method is to present a form of enquiry to each youngster who then proceeds to complete it by himself. It might be better to do without the information rather than to conduct the study in this way.

The atmosphere in which this is all conducted will need to be conducive to the youngster's revealing his true position rather than portraying what he feels we want to know. This is less of a problem than it may seem at a distance. By the time we reach this point, young people are usually taking us very seriously, and in any case are only too interested in their own situation. We shall also need to plan so that the maximum benefit can be drawn from the study, which may be very considerable indeed, for the exercise will usually lead into deep and introspective discussion if the worker is ready to capitalise on the interest raised.

A major decision may have to be taken about whether the group should see the profile of their study. When we first used friendship studies as part of group work we avoided at all costs the youngsters seeing the outcome of their choices. However, as time went by several groups were absolutely insistent that they should see the sociogram and decided from the outset that the study would not be confidential. The discussions that ensued were, on each occasion, so creative that we realised that we could not maintain our previous position. Now each worker approaches this in his own way, and is guided by the stage of development in the group. We feared, in particular, for the youngster who was not well chosen, or who had difficulty in making friendships, but in the event he has usually gained most from the experience, as a result of the group gathering around him in a supportive way. The degree to which the group has already become supportive is probably the key to the decision about whether they are ready to see their own sociometric profile.

The kind of sociogram that may result is illustrated by Figure 2, which shows also the conventional methods of drawing the sociogram. The mechanics are quite simple. The objective of the sociogram is to show the structure of the group and the sub-groups within it, and for this to be clear, as few lines should cross as possible. There is no magic formula for drawing the sociogram; we all have to do it by trial and error. The operation may become more complex if the group is large, especially if there are many interlocking choices. In this case it may be advisable to construct a matrix first: the kind of matrix upon which the sociogram shown here was based is shown in Figure 3. In beginning to draw the sociogram it is usually helpful to start with a person who is well chosen and who is therefore likely to occupy a central position.[1]

[1] For more detailed discussion about sociometry and instructions for preparing a sociogram, see Evans, K. M. (1962) *Sociometry and Education*. London: Routledge and Kegan Paul.

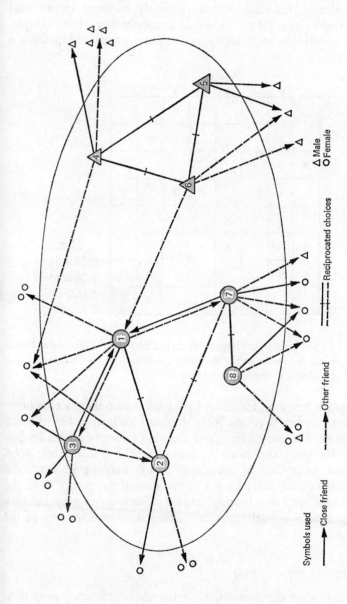

Figure 2 A sociogram of a small group of fourteen–fifteen-year-olds based on a friendship study

Symbols used

▲ Close friend

→ Other friend

╪ Reciprocated choices

△ Male   ○ Female

We cannot deduce from a sociogram based on friendship anything other than the structure of friendships. I find it necessary to emphasise this since, not infrequently, workers try to read from a sociogram information that is just not there. For example, it is not possible to assume any structure of leadership from a

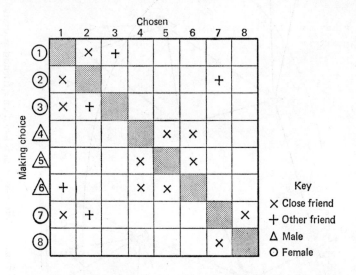

Figure 3　The matrix of the internal choices of the group as depicted in Figure 2: the choices of friends outside the group can be included by numbering each choice and adding to the horizontal axis

sociogram based on friendship, especially since there seems often to be a conflict between friendship and authority. For this we should need a study based on a criterion concerned with leadership. We must also reach in some other way the subtle roles assigned to individual members, which may range from the ideas man or the peace keeper to the idiot of the group. Even the more obvious roles like the clown or scapegoat may be very subtly woven into the general conversation and activity of the group.

Discerning group norms

The way that the group behave together, including even their relationships with one another, will be strongly influenced by the prevailing norms of the group. It is vital for the worker to discern the patterns of normative control as rapidly as possible. The experienced worker will begin to sense the controls from the moment that he makes contact with the group, although the more subtle forms of control may be quite difficult to discern.

There are a number of ways of illuminating the norms influencing a situation. One of them is by direct enquiry, and I am including as Appendix 1a to 1d four forms of enquiry that may be helpful for this purpose. The enquiry has been arranged in four parts, as we have found that it is too big an area to cover on a single occasion. Furthermore, it takes time for a group of young people to become sensitive to the more subtle forms of controls. By beginning with the more concrete manifestations, such as clothes and routines, young people rapidly become much more sophisticated in their understanding, and are then ready to face the more subtle controls that will be influencing their relationships and the content of their communication.

Certain parts of this enquiry are best accomplished through personal conversations with each individual before a general discussion takes place, since we are interested in the differences of perception between the group members as well as the common ground. Other parts are equally suitable for discussion by the whole group. In the event, the worker will need to be guided by what is possible and the kind of contribution that the study can make to the group at its stage of development. He may decide to use the whole enquiry as a basis for a number of exploratory discussions, in which case he will use the forms as an agenda. We have found that we do not need to be furtive about holding an agenda: youngsters usually accept our personal notes of preparation as evidence that we are doing our homework in pursuit of a professional job.

Enquiry form I (pages 186–8) concentrates on the composition of the group, any routine of activity (or inactivity), visible signs of conformity (for example, in clothes), major demands of conformity in behaviour, and on whether the individual's behaviour when with the group differs from his behaviour elsewhere. Although this includes some important areas of information, the enquiry presents, as one of its main purposes, an opportunity for young people to become conscious of the operation of group controls. We find that young people even of moderate intellectual ability, when led into a study of this kind, quickly come to understand group norms as a concept.

The second form of enquiry, included as Appendix 1b (pages 189–90), uses the unfinished sentence technique and is much more open-ended. It is intended to explore the likely or habitual response of the group to a number of situations such as school or work, and to specific people including adults in general, parents, teachers, and members of the opposite sex. It is possible that the response to some questions, such as that about the police, will hardly touch the behaviour of one group but may be central to the consciousness of another. If the initial responses to some of the questions can be followed up by exploratory discussion, it is possible that a great deal of stereotyped and scarcely conscious behaviour will be revealed to both the worker and the group.

The third form of enquiry (pages 191–2) is intended to identify the topics and depth of communication seen by the group as appropriate. The effect of normative influences on overt behaviour are of obvious importance, especially when they lead to mischief and disruption, but it is not so generally realised that the controls on the pattern of communication in a group may be even more important, especially in the way that they limit the development of young people. For example, some groups have been found to outlaw any intimate conversation between their members, and have thus deprived one another of the opportunity for an outlet for pressures that each was carrying. And, at a more mundane level, many groups of young people have limited the actual words that might be used in conversation to a pocket vocabulary. Imagine the plight of the English teacher working with groups like this. The ambitions of the teacher include the extension of vocabulary, fluent use of language, and an active relationship with literature, but any move by one of the young people in this direction will be checked by telling little sanctions, such as 'Swallowed a dictionary?', or 'O.K., Professor!', or merely 'Ponce . . .'.

The forms of enquiry are intended only as a point of entry. If the group have been taken step by step into an understanding of the normative controls operating, they will be ready to explore the deeper implications of what has been revealed. The use of forms of enquiry is not the only way of exploring normative controls. The experienced worker will not in any case wait for a set occasion, but will be picking up events or statements and question the roots of these as they occur. We can also use role-play or socio-drama for this purpose, as is described in Chapter 6.

Roles

Just as the norms of the group may influence the topics and pattern of communication, so they may also strongly influence the pattern of relationships within the group. This may be in a generalised way, as in groups that insist on intimate confidences between members, or alternatively ban any intimate exchanges. Within this general framework, more personal roles will be taken by individuals.

The individual will tend towards certain forms of behaviour that fit comfortably with his personality, there will be a push and pull of individuals accommodating themselves to one another, the individual will settle into an accepted pattern, which will then be structured into the pattern of expectancies of the group. Thus the personal roles of the individual become part of the normative structure of the group, and they place very strong pressures on him to remain within the confines of the role pattern that has been accorded to him.

Some people create for themselves a similar role pattern wherever they go: their range of behaviour may be limited and the group will either have to accord them a compatible role or exclude them completely. Other people may behave differently from one group situation to another. Sometimes people become imprisoned in their role—albeit largely of their own making—from which they are not free to depart.

It is vital that the young people in our groups come to see how they are influencing one another in this way, and gain early insight into the role structure of the group. The fourth form of enquiry, Appendix 1d (pages 192–4), has been designed to begin this process. It focusses on some of the more obvious role-taking in the group, and may help to initiate the examination of the more subtle forms of group expectancies expressed in the behaviour of individual members. This may be further explored through role-play and socio-drama, as well as through discussion and other formal enquiry.[1]

[1] For a concise exploration of roles see Ruddock, R. (1970) *Roles and Relationships*. London: Routledge and Kegan Paul.

Social diagnosis is also social intervention

As Robert Laing has pointed out, in social situations, as distinct from medical situations, it is impossible to carry out diagnosis without influencing the situation that we are diagnosing.[1] It must be clear that if any of the methods of social diagnosis I have suggested above are used, the worker will already have influenced the situation he is examining, sometimes fairly fundamentally. It is important that we should appreciate not only the inevitability of this but also the potential of it. It should also be apparent that diagnosis is not something that is done once and for all. The situation surrounding an individual, and more especially the pattern of interrelationships between a group of people, is always on the move. Diagnosis must therefore be seen as a continuous process; at every stage a new assessment will be necessary which in turn will inform the next move.

For the sake of tidiness in treatment I have devoted separate chapters to diagnosis and techniques of intervention, but not only is this separation artificial, it could also, if carried into practice, limit the fluency of our work. Not only are the methods of diagnosis listed above very effective means of intervention, but many of the techniques listed in Chapter 6, such as role-play or ways of leading to introspective discussion, are equally effective as methods of diagnosis.

Fortunately, the fact that diagnosis and intervention may both arise from the same operation offers great economy, and often the sharper the methods of diagnosis the more they contribute to the on-going experience. Workers who have learnt to make direct and rapid contact sometimes face a hiatus; having surprised themselves by their capacity to make warm and easy contact with young people, they may then find themselves saying, 'Here are the youngsters only too willing to be involved, but what is there *to do*?' They are seeking a context as focus for the group that will be appropriate to the personal needs of the members of the group.

This hiatus can be avoided if the means of making contact are clearly seen as a first step in an on-going diagnosis, for the experience involved in the diagnosis may in itself offer a series of

[1] Laing, R. (1969) *Intervention in Social Situations*. London: Association of Family Caseworkers.

compelling experiences. At first the worker may tend to use methods of diagnosis a little mechanically. It is important that he should see the framework of information, enlightenment and experience as an end to which the actual instruments are a means. When he has built this into a professional framework, he will be able to draw from it more creatively and fluently.

For example, one piece of information he will seek through individual and private conversation; another he will see as an agenda for group discussion; and a third as the subject for a formal enquiry framed in collaboration with the young people concerned.

CHAPTER FIVE

The programme and the experience

Events as experience

It may seem very obvious that the influence upon us of being a member of a group will depend upon the experiences in which we are involved, yet the implications of the statement lead immediately to the examination of the qualities of those experiences. Experience arises out of events. A conversation between two people is an event or a series of events; even lack of activity may be seen as an event. Most 'activities' are a series of events and may have a variety of experience within them. Lack of events may induce ennui; a surfeit of them may cause confusion. A repetitive cycle of events will bring little challenge and change, for we shall have well-rehearsed responses for such situations. If we are wanting to induce growth and change, we must clearly bring young people to new experiences, and probably of a particular kind.

In a group situation the impact of activity reaches the individual in several ways. The events in which he is involved have their intrinsic quality and his personal participation in them will bring a direct impact upon him. For example, there is a certain experience arising from covering an area of paper with a single colour, which is different from creating form and pattern with a variety of colours, and that is a very different experience again from interviewing a stranger in the street. An important part of the experience is embedded in the approach to the activity, such as how much inventiveness and self-determination it calls from us. In so far as education is concerned with experience, the approach may be an important part of the content.

When a group of people engage in an activity as a joint undertaking, an additional dimension is added to the experience in terms of the influence of the activity on the interpersonal contacts, but here again the experience depends very much upon the way the activity is approached. For example, the appointed leader may easily short-circuit much of the potential experience for the members by taking all the major responsibilities himself, thus saving them the need to cope with one another in decision-taking and action.

A group of people will usually tend to seek an equilibrium in their relationships with one another in which everyone knows where he stands, and will thus settle down to expected, repetitive and sometimes stereotype roles. Any activity that is conducted within this framework tends to be subjected to an automatic and unconscious process of selection to see that it fits the existing expectancies and relationships within the group. We may wish to disturb the equilibrium so that the members of the group may break free from unhelpful stereotypes, or extend their experience by assuming new roles. This will probably necessitate gaining acceptance of new kinds of activity, but the way the group approaches the activity, and in particular the amount of responsibility carried by the group for organising its own affairs, is also very important. And different kinds of activity will once again induce very different kinds of experiences, particularly in terms of the degree to which the members must cope with new situations, with one another, and with people outside their own group.

The experience within the activity

I must be cautious in the use of the word 'activity' since this may be interpreted, particularly in the world of youth work, as an identifiable pursuit, which may be taught or led as a specialism. I am using 'activity' here more as a generic term, implying anything that gives rise to a series of events. In wishing to accelerate experience and growth we shall need to study the effects of different kinds of activity. The proposition that different activities have different kinds of experience inherent in them leads to a vital study for the group worker. There has been very little exact study on this subject, and what has been done has tended not to distinguish between the intrinsic quality of the activity and the pattern of interaction and other interpersonal features to which it gives rise.[1]

[1] Davies, B. (1969) 'Activity in Youth Work'. In *Youth Review*, No. 14.

It is sometimes suggested that whatever the artist draws or paints is a self-portrait, or that it is possible to diagnose personality from movement. Does this mean that, since our efforts in these fields express our personalities, if we can learn new approaches in them then our personality may change a little as well? Some of the attention given in traditional youth work to outdoor pursuits seemed to be based on this assumption, and has been severely criticised for it. It is interesting to note that several recent studies of the effect of Outward Bound courses seem to suggest that there may, after all, be some carry-over of effect from one department of life to another.[1]

Whether we recognise it or not, most of us are very formative in the activities adopted by the groups with which we work: witness the frequency with which a group catches the worker's enthusiasm for sailing, drama, travel, rock climbing, or whatever it may be. The group worker will need to be judicious and deliberate in leading his group to a new context. For example, how are we to address ourselves to the all too frequent condition arising out of a low sense of social worth? The pat answer is that anything that brings success may boost the youngster's sense of importance, but we will meet youngsters who are unlikely to be good at any of the traditional exploits that are seen as achievements.

It is worth asking ourselves what it is in success that so boosts the ego; is it largely the approbation that it brings from others, the reflection of one's worth in other people's eyes which brings also an increase in status in our own? Is it not possible to approach this increase of status, this greater sense of worth to other people, in a more direct and certain way? A low sense of social worth is sometimes allied, in a particular youngster, with an inability to love or to accept love. Yet we have found that many of these youngsters are capable of compassion, as long as they meet something sufficiently compelling to touch them deeply.

Youngsters suffering from these disabilities have been stirred to a new level of social competence and feeling by finding

[1] Fletcher, B. A. (1970) *Outward Bound*. Bristol: School of Education, University of Bristol.

Payne, J., Drummond, A. W. and Lunghi, M. (1970) 'Changes in Self Concepts of School Leavers who Participated in an Arctic Expedition'. *British Journal of Educational Psychology*, Vol. 40, Part 2, pages 211–15.

themselves of some value and service to other people, especially when they have been stirred by the plight of people worse off than themselves. Their response to this kind of experience can be quite dramatic. They can be elated by the feeling that they can be of service to others, and that others are prepared to express their need of them. Appropriate experience and activity will often take us outside the boundaries of tiaditional subjects and activities.

The activity and the approach

I have already suggested that the impact of the activity may depend as much upon the approach as upon the activity itself. Take, for example, some service to old people. It is possible for the worker to approach this by explaining fully to the youngster what is needed, producing the job of service that is waiting to be done, organising the occasion and allocating duties, merely requiring the youngsters to perform some practical task. In this way he will keep down to a minimum the awkwardness of the parties having to cope with one another. This is the way that so much community service by young people is actually organised.

Compare this approach with one that encourages the youngster first to discover the need for himself, to decide what the response to the need should be, to organise his contribution for himself as far as he is able, and to address himself to the real need in collaboration with the person he is helping. I have known people to be extremely critical of the second approach because of the 'inefficiency' of the operation, and because the amount of 'work' done was less than was thought appropriate, as if the whole purpose of the project was to achieve a certain level of productivity. This surely ignores the major question of what kind of experience is inherent in the operation, both for the youngsters and the old people whom they are helping. In any case it is quite possible that the need has been wrongly diagnosed: for the old person to have someone to converse with, to sense a personal concern in the youngster, might approach more nearly his real need than having his sticks chopped up. Just as we are concerned that the youngster should derive a higher level of self-esteem from the experience, so we would hope that we would in no way reduce the sense of self-reliance and self-esteem in the old person. Why should the old people not also derive satisfaction and personal growth from their part in the exchange?

I shall be returning to this theme when considering action research in greater detail in Chapter 6.

In teaching and youth work we are continually neutralising a whole world of experience for young people by abrogating unto ourselves so many of the functions that might confront them with new situations, and the need to cope with outside forces. I would invite the reader who is a teacher, youth worker, or in other ways concerned with the development of other people, to cast his mind back to the events of his last occasion with them: did you perform functions that saved the young people concerned having to cope with certain things for themselves? We may be able to argue that they would not in any case be capable of coping with these functions, but this is convincing only as long as we have a clear strategy for building their competence step by step, and an unerring policy of not doing anything that they can do for themselves.

Personal–task continuum

Activities and events may also be described in terms of the way that they lead either into or away from intimate exchange. It is possible to conceive a continuum of events from those that inevitably involve exchanges at a personal and intimate level, to others conducted at a completely impersonal or task level.[1] Any exchange between two people may take place at a notional point on this continuum as suggested by Figure 4.

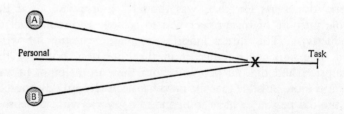

Figure 4 Two people (A and B) usually communicate with one another about something (X) that is mainly or in part outside their intimate selves. As the kind of topic changes, X might be at any part of the personal–task continuum

[1] Button, L. (1967) *Some Experiments in Informal Group Work.* (Pages 14–17.) Swansea: University College of Swansea, Department of Education.

We tend to find it much easier to cope with other people at a task or functional level and this is particularly true of those who have difficulty with intimate relationships. It is as if we seek safety in matter-of-fact areas of conversation and exchange. In our group work we may wish to bring people into contact with one another at a more personal level, and we may well find that group activity at a task or functional level will defeat our purpose by offering a ready retreat to safe areas of action and conversation.

This is part of the rationale behind the use of T-groups for therapeutic purposes. The group, held by the influence of an inactive leader, find themselves without a task in the sense of something outside themselves. Being without a task to perform, the group do not need to structure themselves into a working body, and are held in a state of flux and uncertainty, in which roles may change, sometimes with considerable rapidity. This situation may be found uncomfortable, but most of the members of the group gradually acclimatise themselves to it. As time passes it becomes appropriate for the group to talk at a personal level, and the attempts to introduce a task are then seen as inappropriate.[1]

Towards a model

A good deal of attention has been given in Chapters 3 and 4 to the contribution of interviews and other contacts between the worker and individual young people, and it may be appropriate at this stage to emphasise that the main tool for the work is the group itself. This does not mean that our objectives reside in the progress of the group as a corporate entity, though this may have its importance; our objectives are about the development of individual people and the group is a means to this. It may be helpful at this stage if we could construct a model for the work, a coherent scheme that will help us discern the interconnections between one action and another. In Figure 5 (see page 75) I have

---

[1] For a brief analysis of the T-group situation, see Button, L. (1971) *Discovery and Experience*. London: Oxford University Press. (Page 142.)
For a fuller account, see:
Bion, W. R. (1961) *Experiences in Groups*. London: Tavistock Press.
Ottaway, A. K. C. (1966) *Learning through Group Experience*. London: Routledge and Kegan Paul. Richardson, E. (1967) *Group Study for Teachers*. London: Routledge and Kegan Paul.

suggested the elements of such a model and the interplay between those elements.

Expressions like adjustment, attitude change, and personal development seem sometimes to conjure up a picture of paternal or big brother interest. Similarly the mention of therapy some-times induces, in both trainee workers and bystanders, pictures of surgical incisions, or of giving a machine a wrench with a spanner. It is most important that we should appreciate, first, the organic nature of change and growth, and, second, the need for the client to be in a central position in decision-taking. This brings us to the very core of our work: that the ultimate self-reliance and self-determination of the youngster, and in the meantime the growing autonomy of the group, is central to the objectives of our work as suggested in Figure 5 (page 75). If we can keep this in the forefront of our minds we may be less tempted to induce an acceptance of our own standards, or to use the group as a boost to our own ego. Our diagnosis needs to be a shared diagnosis, with the youngster playing a central role in the investigation of his situation, his problems, and his own responses. Only in this way can he be in the position to take informed decisions about his own actions.

The approaches of the group worker are becoming increasingly sophisticated and influential, and could be misused. There is a fine line between helping and manipulating, and the group worker's methods are equally available to the professional persuader. It is in part with the purpose of protecting young people and ourselves from our professional enthusiasm that we must keep central to our ambitions the growing autonomy of the individual.

We are in an age of increasing choice, of individual morality, and of a democratic life in the sense that we are each of us freer to decide how we should behave. This adds greatly to the need for a capacity for personal judgement and action, and the pressures that emanate from powerful commercial interests add urgency to this need. Part of the deliberate purpose of the worker will be to help the youngsters build a basis for that independent action. In this context it may be well to remind ourselves that personal autonomy means that we must also be in control of our own impulses.

It is possible for the group worker and social worker to take the respect for the personal autonomy of the client to absurd lengths, sometimes under the banner of being 'non-judgemental'. Does this mean also that we must be 'non-influencing'? If we take any hand in people's lives we must necessarily be influencing them; our position is one of inescapable leadership, which we shall exercise as surely by our inactivity as by our positive intervention. Are we to be so neutral that, for example, we shall not attempt to steer young people away from anti-social activity which bears directly on their neighbours? And when we see that a youngster's unhappiness arises from an inability to get along with his peers, are we not to act upon this insight which may have been denied to the youngster himself?

In-group and outside experience

Many counselling and therapeutic groups are based entirely on the conversation between the members of the group, stimulated by what they bring into the group from their daily lives, and in some cases the counsellor or therapist plays a neutral and fairly inactive role. The interplay of a small group that meets regularly and is supportive of its members, may be a very rewarding experience in itself; but we have come to see that to limit the experience in a group to what arises from the conversation between them may just not reach the kind of experience that is vital to certain of the members.

For example, one of our collaborators brought together a group of apprentices as an experiment in group work in industry. Although the conversation in the group overflowed into their normal time at work, there was little in the programme beyond the contact and conversation with one another. The boys gained a great deal from their experience, and the manager was so impressed by their obvious development that he suggested that it might be helpful if the group could make themselves responsible for receiving the new annual intake of apprentices. But when the occasion arrived the boys sheepishly gathered into a corner, and showed themselves quite incapable of receiving the newcomers: one of the things they had not been able to learn in their closed group was how to meet strangers.

This is a very simple illustration of the limitations of the closed conversation group. It is usually necessary to seek certain activity that takes the members beyond the confines of the group in order to offer them opportunities for vital experience, and to feed new impetus into the relationships within the group. I shall call this 'outside experience' as distinct from 'in-group experience' arising from the interchange between the members of the group (see Figure 5, page 75). We are then faced immediately by the question: what kind of experience based on what kind of activity? The intrinsic experience inherent in the activity will need to be appropriate to the needs of the individual members of the group, and the activity should also stir the group as a whole in ways that are helpful to its members.

For illustration I will revert to the example of interviewing a stranger in the street as part of a longer on-going project. The personal experiences reaching the group member as a result of this will include: daring to tackle the stranger who is preoccupied with his own concerns and does not expect to be approached in this way; marshalling the necessary explanation and putting the other person at his ease; conducting himself in an acceptable and attractive way; ordering his procedure and maintaining the flow of the exchanges; expressing appreciation and making the other person feel the encounter was rewarding. The experience accruing to the group, working as a team, will depend upon how the project is being approached, and may include: envisaging and debating the project; formulating an enquiry (with all the discussion, sifting of suggestion, and the allocation of the work entailed); rehearsing the approach to interviewing, each facing his own fears of rejection and encouraging colleagues in their efforts; leaving the other members of the group in order each to undertake his personal share of interviewing (which may be a major step with a tight group who always hang around together); and processing the material. The corporate experience of the group so much depends upon the approach of the worker; some youth workers and teachers seem under an inner compulsion to assume all the organising roles themselves.

A project that includes interviewing strangers in the street might or might not be an appropriate experience for any particular group of youngsters, and the worker will always have to judge whether to encourage his groups to seek this or that experience. The proper basis for this judgement is his diagnosis both of the position of the individual and of the condition of the group as a whole. For example, if the group is one that never separates, which ties each of its members as if they were on a ball and chain, it might be quite a challenging experience for the members of the group to undertake an assignment on their own or with a single partner.

In considering the kind of experience that we might encourage young people to seek, we need to bear in mind these two principles: first, that it should approach as directly and economically as possible the heart of the youngster's need; and, second, that experience should come in the right order, so that having assimilated one experience he is reasonably well prepared to meet something a little more testing. On the worker's part, there will need to be careful thought and planning at each stage, inspired by a long-term strategy.

The exploration of relationships

It is common in therapeutic or developmental group work for the group to discuss the relationship between its members. In fact, in some forms of group therapy and social work in groups, discussion between the members about their feelings, both in general and for one another, is the major part of the process.[1] This kind of discussion is an important part also of the style of group work which we have been developing, but we seek additional experience that is likely to stimulate within the group exchanges of a more personal nature.

It seems that without something to stir the group and the equilibrium of their relationships, much of the raw material for therapy may be lacking. A certain element of stress would seem to be a prerequisite of personal movement and development. If, therefore, we can encourage the group to undertake some activity that demands new roles and interpersonal relationships, and stirs emotionally the individual members, it is possible that we may be able to accelerate the process of development and therapy.[2] The project hinted at above, especially if it is approached through action research, will involve a group in a whole range of new functions, and the members will therefore need to accept new roles. It may also greatly stir each member's compassion, and so stir latent emotions within them, and is therefore likely to

[1] McCullough, M. C. and Ely, P. (1968) *Social Work with Groups*. London: Routledge and Kegan Paul.
[2] Button, L. (1971) *Discovery and Experience*. London: Oxford University Press. (Chapter X.)

produce a good deal of raw material leading to the examination of relationships.

This section is advisedly headed 'exploration' rather than 'discussion' of relationships. We are faced with the difficulty that the same project is intended to help a group of people whose individual needs may be different. To some extent each will draw selectively from the same experience, according to what fits his own position, but it is possible for the group, by showing care and thought for individual members, to increase considerably the differentiation of experience arising out of the same programme. It is not only a matter of discussing relationships, it is also one of role-taking, and individual members may be encouraged to take on the roles that most fit their needs. As a worker in a school reported:

> The group then turned to a discussion of Terry's behaviour. His role in life, it seemed, was that of the scapegoat, and as they examined it more closely they grasped its significance. They seemed fascinated by the idea of personal roles, and by the possibility of changing roles, particularly Terry's role. They set about considering what they could do to help.

It is really very impressive to discover how clear-sighted young people can be, and how much help they can give one another after deliberate thought. For example, a violent gang knowingly assigned new and creative roles to their erstwhile leader in violence. This required a conscious decision on their part because he was less secure in these new roles, which would almost certainly have been filled by another member of the group who had much more social competence. In a similar way, other groups have taken in hand a member who always behaved to them and to his other peers in ways that would earn his rejection, and have encouraged him to try new approaches and take new roles.

Expression of feeling and introspective discussion

Once a group of youngsters have been stimulated emotionally and have begun to examine their own relationships, they will very soon be looking into themselves. This process may fall into two fairly distinct parts: first, the members may express feelings that do not easily find expression; and, second, they may discuss objectively what they are feeling, and what might be the roots of those feelings. For example, a youngster might be very moved whilst confessing to the group his feelings of timidity and shyness; this may be the beginning of a second phase: the objective discussion of these feelings and their origins, coupled with efforts by the young person concerned, supported by the other members of the group, to acclimatise himself to increasingly demanding situations.

In this kind of discussion youngsters may learn things that they did not know about themselves, in spite of having lived with these characteristics for, say, fifteen years. For example, a youngster who had earned for himself the reputation of being a 'creep' by continually referring to his teachers for reassurance was quite unaware of the fact that he was behaving any differently from other people. When this was revealed, and his erstwhile critics saw the real situation, they immediately closed round him and supported him in his efforts to change his behaviour. In a supportive group situation, an individual youngster may be able to take from his peers enlightenment that he would reject from a parent or other adult in authority, or, for that matter, from his peers outside this warm, objective and controlled situation.

In the next chapter I shall discuss more fully the contribution of intimate conversation to development and therapy; at this stage I want merely to draw the distinction between the exploration of relationships and introspective discussion. If we grasp these two aspects of the work as separate concepts—though they may well flow into one another—it helps us to lead into either or both if we consider it desirable. The discussion of relationships may be about overt behaviour as well as feelings for one another; introspective discussion is about internal emotional states that underlie behaviour, including our feelings about ourselves.

It is not difficult to lead into introspective discussion: it is largely a matter of conversation at that level being accepted as appropriate, which in turn is bound up with the normative controls of the group. Group norms can outlaw certain levels or topics of conversation as well as make them legitimate. Close friendship often has this quality within it, of an outlet for confession and intimate conversation, though we have discovered in our research that some friendships have become crystallised with very limited scope for intimate exchanges. Workers often fear frank talk in their groups, but many have reported that their fears were proved groundless:

> They suddenly decided to say frankly how they saw one another. I feared that all my work so far was going to be destroyed by this conversation, but I have to admit that at that moment the group became more supportive than they had ever been before, and (they) have continued at a new level of intimacy and support.

The development of introspective discussion can be accelerated in a number of ways, notably by the group becoming involved in an introspective study, opportunities for which are inherent in a number of the diagnostic procedures outlined above. For example, it is not difficult to build on the discussions that take place about friendship when a friendship study is undertaken, and this is one of the ways in which the partnership in diagnosis between the worker and young people can be so helpful. In the next chapter I shall be suggesting a number of ways in which we may be able to initiate introspective studies and stimulate introspective discussion.

Strategy

In Figure 5 I have attempted to bring together in a coherent framework the element of group work that I have described. The growing autonomy of the group and of the individual is shown as being central to the whole purpose. The in-group experience, the benefit that arises from being a member of an intimate, supportive and objective group, changes in quality as the group develops. The outside experience to which the group expose themselves will feed immediately into the quality of the in-group experience as well as into the personal experiences of each individual. If the outside experience is wisely chosen, it is likely to stir the members of the group and will therefore help to stimulate the exploration of relationships and introspective discussion. These two elements will feed into one another, and enhance further the quality of the experience involved in being a member of the group. If the group can be encouraged to undertake some kind of introspective study, this will immediately stimulate their introspective discussion and probably the exploration of relationships as well.

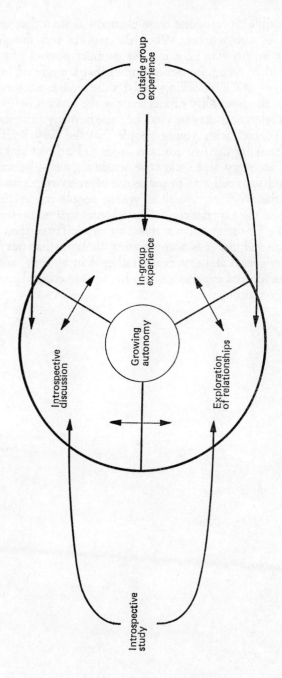

Figure 5 The interlocking parts of group work which reinforce one another

It is possible to recognise these elements as steps that may be influenced by the worker. When the worker sees the process analytically in this way he is in a far stronger position, for he is better placed to recognise opportunities that are offered to him. The elements are interlocking and reinforce one another, and this adds to the possibility of accelerating the process.

That acceleration may be vital, because in many situations the length of contact with young people may be very brief. The process of making the first contacts needs to be direct and rapid, our work at every stage must be sensitive, well-planned and incisive, and we need also to make use of every opportunity to accelerate the work as rapidly as young people can acclimatise themselves to the experience. We have found that youngsters can usually take in their stride a speed of work faster than most workers can induce. It is a comforting thought that our work proceeds by events and experience rather than by time, and that ten minutes' crucial experience may have more effect than hours of safe conversation.

CHAPTER SIX

Repertoire of techniques

Group work has both benefited and also suffered from sharing skills and theoretical concepts with counselling, psycho-therapy, other forms of social work and some approaches to teaching. There tend to be various schools of thought. An approach may be described as 'non-directive', 'client-based', 'group-based', 'psycho-analytical', or 'behaviourist', and there may be pre-conceptions that inspire but also limit each of these approaches.

In developing our own work we have tended to be rather more pragmatic, and have seized upon anything that seems to be helpful. As we have explored the effect of what we are doing, we have attempted to add to a conceptual framework and to a repertoire of techniques. As a result, our approach has become many-sided, and we have found that one element interlocks with, and reinforces or releases, another. We have come to see the experience that reaches young people as central to the whole process. Some kinds of experiences not only have value in themselves, but also trigger off a series of other and sometimes deeper experiences. In general, the tougher the problem the greater will be the need for depth in the experience of the group.

The client as his own therapist

One of the major purposes of our work is to ensure that young people should be better able to help themselves after their contact with us has ended; and as it is also part of our ambition to help establish a caring community, it is just as important that they should learn how to help and support other people. To this end we take young people into our confidence in every possible way, so that they may come to share some of our functions. We will involve them as fully as possible in our diagnosis, and we will tend to work through open-ended statements, inviting them to come inside our thinking.

It is very impressive to see how rapidly young people will share the group worker's role. Individual youngsters may sometimes lead a phase of questioning of one of their colleagues, and as they learn how to recognise the need for help and to offer help, this soon begins to flow beyond the confines of the group. Many become involved in supportive roles to people outside their group, making use of the group for encouragement and advice in what they are attempting.

Reg and Alec expressed some anxiety about a girl in their class at the Tech., who seemed to be lonely, whose work was going downhill, and who was becoming the butt of the same teacher who had been attacking Reg. They decided that the least they could do was to offer her kindness and support, and they might even be able to do something about the growing pressure from the teacher. After all, their conversations with him had already changed his whole approach to Reg.

When a group of youngsters reach this stage, support for one another through discussion and action may continue outside the group meetings. The worker needs to be aware of this possibility, for the situation may have changed in the intervening period since he was last with them.

It is not only that the members of the group may become partners in the diagnosis of their situation: they may also express views about the effectiveness of the worker's action. Both in our research and in our development of methods of group work we have had reason to be very grateful to the many youngsters who have offered us new points of enlightenment. It is especially in laying strategy that the youngsters may share the responsibility and the decision.

Janet, feeling the support of the group and having been stirred by the discussion, described in a moving though faltering statement the depth of her shyness, which at times brought her a feeling of nausea at the prospect of meeting new people. Already by reason of her statement her position had changed. With great sensitivity the group discussed her feelings with her, and considered with her what they could do to help.

A number of Janets have demonstrated that with the help of their peers, they can make very considerable progress; and the rest of the group find the experience of offering such help elevating and rewarding. Not only does it boost their own egos that they can help in this way, but it also demonstrates to them the scope there might be for their own development.

It should be second nature to the group worker always to put the client in the strong position. I mean by this that, at every opportunity, he will feed to the youngster the necessity for initiative, especially in his relationship with the worker. Involving the youngster in an examination of his own problems (as in action research, which is described below) typifies this approach, as does education through discovery in the teaching world, for if we are proceeding on the discoveries made by young people, it immediately increases the strength of their position. Although we may help them to explore the full significance of their discoveries, they and they alone can tell us what they have uncovered.

When applied to teaching, the experience provides much more than a store of knowledge: we are nurturing a habit of self-help and self-reliance in study, and we are likely also to be feeding rather than satisfying the student's curiosity. By using similar methods in the training of professional workers, for example, teachers, group workers, or social workers, we can ensure that a wide range of skills are practised by the trainee at the same time as he assumes an independence of action. In group work we may face an apparent paradox when the worker takes a very active role in order to induce self-reliance in young people. The worker's activity consists largely of encouraging them to assume roles of action and initiative, as a result of which they may grow in competence and independence.

In the leader–follower relationship, every time the follower initiates action for the leader he shortens the distance between them in terms of authority. When there is something to be done the worker will encourage the group to identify what is needed, suggest how it should be done, and arrange for certain of its number to take it on. He will not himself do anything that he can encourage some other member of the group to do. There will be some functions that the worker may have to undertake, in which case he will consult the group about how the members would like these tasks to be accomplished.

Sometimes it is difficult to engage young people in active

participation, though this is usually as a result of timidity rather than unwillingness to cooperate. We find that this situation can often be changed quite quickly by proceeding through small working parties. I shall be describing this technique in Chapter 9[1] in the context of work with larger groups, but it is equally effective and sometimes very necessary when working with small groups of, say, only eight or ten.

Group support

I have already used the expression 'supportive group' a number of times, and there is no doubt that the support that is offered to young people both by the group worker and by their peers in the group is an extremely important part of their experience.

A supportive atmosphere often causes people to be much more open to change. In ordinary life, when we tell people what we think of them we may have very little impact on them; our urging them to change seems to build up its own resistance. In a supportive situation, the person who is the subject of criticism may be able to allow himself to become associated with that criticism. It is as if he crosses the frontier, and stands with his colleagues looking in on himself objectively. It is not a neutral situation and often not a comfortable one, for the person concerned may be considering some fairly trenchant statements about himself.

On many occasions supportiveness will grow naturally out of the group's being together and doing things together, but at other times we shall be wishing to hasten its growth. It will be helpful if we can foresee steps that we can take in order to increase the level of support. It may seem almost a truism to suggest that supportiveness is unlikely to arise unless there is a need for it—that the support for someone engaged in intimate discussion may arise out of the very fact that intimate conversation is taking place. The supportive response to a charged and difficult situation may be immediate. This runs counter to the view sometimes held by group workers that they should not lead their groups to intimate conversation until a supportive situation has been created. It also points the distinction between supportive and 'cosy' situations. Many supportive situations are anything but

[1] See *Socratic group discussion*, pages 156-61.

cosy, and groups are often at their most supportive when the going is hardest.

Much depends upon the worker's skill in leading the conversation into more intimate exchanges: he must be sensitive to the emotional tone underlying what is being said. And the manner of his leadership has immediate effect. At times we may find ourselves drawing attention to the emotional pressures being experienced by a number of the group, and we will wish to do it in a way that implies our own concern. A group usually catches the worker's tone. It is important that the worker should be seen as offering a warm and obviously caring form of leadership, rather than the neutral and somewhat enigmatic position taken up by some workers.

Thus the worker may share with the group his problem of creating a helpful and supportive climate and if this becomes one of the acknowledged aims of the group, the members may move in this direction quite rapidly. The need for support can readily be identified during role-play, for the people who reveal their own emotional position through the parts that they play usually draw the whole group's sympathy and encouragement. This can be of special importance when working with larger groups, in which offering statements, or taking initiative, can be that much more challenging. In this kind of situation it can be profitable to lead directly and openly into discussions about the daring that is required to play one's part, and about the ways in which members can offer support to one another.

Physical contact

There is little doubt that warmth and support can sometimes be induced through physical contact. As I mentioned in Chapter 2, it is possible that the need for physical contact, so vital to the infant, never really leaves us, though its expression is regulated by convention in most communities and severely limited in some. In recent years considerable attention has been given in some forms of group work to the release of feeling through physical contact.[1] This has been variously described as, for example, 'sensitivity training',[2] or 'encounter groups', although Carl

[1] Schutz, W. C. (1973) *Joy*. Harmondsworth: Penguin Books.
[2] McGuinness, T. (1970) 'Sensitivity Training in a Partly Dehumanized Environment'. *Marriage Guidance*, September 1970.

Rogers uses the term encounter group to describe the much more general experience of a small group of people meeting regularly in a supportive face-to-face situation.[1]

Many of the situations described by group workers who encourage physical contact are of groups brought together specifically for this purpose. The experience is usually relatively brief, there is little by way of diagnosis, and the experience is seen as being complete in itself without any follow-up. When we first tentatively introduced this kind of experience into our own work, we did so cautiously and judiciously. Many of the groups described in the literature were quite different from our own—for example, the situations described by McGuinness were with students, and probably mainly middle-class students at that, whereas even the taking of the hand may be a very strange experience for many working-class youngsters. The worker will need to assess his situation carefully. Many workers are answerable to surrounding establishment and community groups who could be outraged by something that they saw as wildly unconventional, and they must therefore judge carefully their own social situations. It is not that they would wish to be social conformists, but at a minimum they do not want to be stopped from doing a useful job.

The climate has, in fact, changed very rapidly and we have found that most groups are prepared to accept some kinds of physical contact as being appropriate to the group meetings. For example, one street group of working-class youngsters came to see hand taking as a symbol of their meeting, especially when new members joined the group, even if this occurred in the open street. We have successfully used some kind of physical contact as part of the programme of a wide variety of groups, ranging from club groups and street groups to large groups of less able fourth-formers and groups of sixth-formers in school.

We tend to use physical contact in an organic way by weaving it into a programme of experience, where it contributes appropriately and at the right time to a longer-term experience, rather than as a separate exercise as it is often practised. For example, it may form part of the introductory experience of a group, even of people who have known one another for a number of years. A phase of this kind might begin with taking the hand of each

[1] Rogers, C. (1970) *Encounter Groups.* Harmondsworth: Penguin Books.

person in the room, followed by eye contact at the same time as taking the hand. The members of the group might be invited to explore the hands of the other people in the room, so that later they can recognise the hands with their eyes closed. This can be done by arranging an inner and outer circle, the inner circle stationary with eyes closed and the outer circle moving round until given the word to offer their hands to the person in front of them. After a time the inner and outer circle can change places. The experience can be treated partly as a game, though the members of the group usually grasp the significance of the experience quite rapidly.

There is likely to be an initial period of awkwardness, and the whole sequence may need to be fairly strongly led. Any embarrassment usually passes quite quickly, most groups soon begin to enjoy the experience, and a feeling of warmth may grow rapidly. Indeed, an expansiveness may be engendered that overflows into other facets of life. Much will depend upon the way in which the occasion is led. For example, we may wish to focus attention on what we are expressing through our hands, or encourage members of the group to try to express their support for one another through hand taking and eye contact. Support may also be expressed when we invite pairs to lead one another as if one of them were blind. Are they making sure that their partner is both feeling secure and is conscious of their concern?

Certain members of the group may be taking part in this activity reluctantly, and we must be ready to enable them to express their unwillingness without loss of face, and possibly to cope with their criticism. This is important because the participants have not come specifically to engage in physical contact, as in the case of a pre-announced 'encounter group' which is largely self-selective for this reason. It is often those who find it most difficult at first who are later most vocal about the value of the experience to them.

If we are using physical contact as means of introduction, it can, with considerable profit, be woven into exploratory discussion. For example, we may ask each person to find as a partner someone whom he does not know very well or would like to know better. The conversation might take this form:

'Take your partner aside and engage him in a personal conversation. Help him to tell you about himself.'

D

After a few minutes' discussion, it may be helpful to break in with:

> 'How good are we at listening? Listening is an active process and our responses should help the other person to identify the experiences and feelings that he would like to share with us.'

After each pair has had time to converse at a fairly personal level, a change of partner could be suggested:

> 'Now would each pair find another pair? Would you each introduce yourself to the other pair, and do this in the first person but in the character of your partner. "I am Jane Brown . . .".'

There is a lot of experience to be drawn from an event of this kind—for example, the real meaning of empathy. After a period of sorting out, when the first person will have begun his account of what he has learnt about his partner, we may feel that we can interrupt with:

> 'Let's pause for a moment. Are we really in the shoes of our partner? How strong a capacity for empathy have we? Are we that other person and are we experiencing some of the feelings that he or she has shared with us? Feel yourself into the skin of your partner.'

It is after attempting to feel themselves into the other person's position that many participants realise that they have heard from their partner but have not understood or empathised.

There are a considerable number of strands to a single experience of this kind. The freedom of personal expression grows very rapidly. Each person feels involved with a number of other people and as a result very much more at ease. And many have become remarkably well acquainted with one another, which serves as a point of departure for later discussions. The level of support may have increased considerably and at a very early stage a standard of intercommunication has been set which has long-term effects on the exchanges of the group. In, say, a little more than an hour the group will have come to understand certain concepts such as support, active listening, levels and kinds of communication, and the meaning of empathy. Some will also have increased their sensitivity to other people, which will carry over to situations outside the group situation.

Those longer-term effects are often quite evident. A worker describing an occasion with a group of fifteen-year-old working class youngsters reported:

They were obviously deeply interested and very sensitive in the way that they were hearing from one another. Suddenly Sean surprised us all by bursting into tears: something we had been talking about had obviously touched a cord in him. He told us amid his tears about family difficulties with one of his brothers for whom he obviously felt strongly. He had not told any of his friends about this before, and it was obviously something of a family skeleton. The group reacted to his tears immediately. Linda moved across and took his hand, and Joan drew up her chair a little closer on the other side. Harry moved round behind him and put a little weight on his right shoulder, whilst Ralph delivered a series of slow and gentle biffs to his other shoulder. It was an extremely supportive moment. I have little doubt that last week's experience of physical contact was having its effect, for the natural mores of young people in this district would normally have prevented a display of support through physical contact.

Action research

I have already suggested that the approach adopted for any plan of action may be as important a part of the experience as the activity involved; indeed, it may make it a different kind of activity. Take, for example, community service as one of the activities to be undertaken by a group of young people. Through action research the worker can lead the group to discover the need, to prepare to meet the need, to perform the service that seems to be required, and to reassess the situation in readiness for renewed action.

We call this approach 'action research' because through their enquiry the participants already begin to affect the situation they are examining. Their discoveries also have a strong impact on them, and stir in them a determination to take some action about the situation they have uncovered. The whole process induces objectivity, and often compassion, so that the situation is approached realistically rather than in a sentimental or glamorised way. Action research differs from exact research since it leads the enquirer into becoming enmeshed with what he is examining, whereas the academic researcher is more detached and takes his findings away from the situation.

It is important that we should be able to see action research as a series of developing steps.

SEIZING UPON A CONTEXT

Anything that stirs the members of a group may serve as a context for action research. It will often have its origins in the personal or intimate exchanges within the group. For example, a sociometric study of the group has led quite naturally to a discussion of friendship, and, as it so often does, to the expression of quite strong feelings about loneliness. The group worker has encouraged the group to focus on loneliness, and they have asked themselves whether there are lonely people around them. This has caught the compassion of some and the interests of others, and they may soon begin to look outside their group, either at their school or club, or at their own neighbourhood. One or two members may well be able to cite cases where they believe loneliness exists, but they may not at this stage have seen their own ability to do anything about it, or their feelings may not yet be strong enough to carry them into positive action. They may, however, feel it worth while to make a few tentative enquiries.

PILOT ENQUIRY

Is there, in fact, a problem worthy of the group's attention? A pilot enquiry might be accomplished by a concise framework of questions addressed either to a number of people at hand or to a specific class of people. Alternatively it could take the form of informal consultation with knowledgeable people. In the case of the suggested interest in loneliness, a short preliminary enquiry might be addressed to parents and neighbours, or several informed people, such as a welfare worker, a clergyman, or a doctor, might be invited to meet the group.

We need to exercise some care when arranging for visitors to meet the group. When young people are engaged in action research they should remain central to the action, and the purpose of receiving visitors is to hold them in a dialogue, not to hear a speech. Preparing the youngsters for a dialogue is usually not difficult, but the visitor also will need to be prepared. In fact it is usually more difficult to prepare the visitor, for he may expect to give a speech. Here the roles are different; the youngsters are the enquirers and the visitor is a resource person rather than a specialist speaker. Young people rapidly become skilled at this kind of exchange and may be critical of the adult who cannot take his place in a dialogue.

MAIN ENQUIRY

By this time the imagination and concern of most young people is stirred, they are taking themselves seriously and are ready to undertake a further enquiry or survey that will bring them face-to-face with people who suffer real loneliness. All the time the worker will be helping them to build up their confidence and competence. Step by step they will have cleared their minds through discussion and role-play; they will have consulted peers, parents and neighbours; they will have laid some plans for their own further enlightenment, received visitors and held them in a dialogue; they will have conceived the possibility of a survey and have formulated their enquiry, and have organised the survey that they are to undertake. All this may have taken place during a very short time, which in itself is a measure of the speed at which they may grow in competence.

The purpose of the main enquiry is to reveal the extent of the problem, to ascertain whether any help or change in the situation is needed, and to judge how far the action required is within the competence of the young people concerned. There is need for some caution on the part of the worker. Action research is intended to lead directly into action in order to help deal with the situation that has been uncovered. It is therefore most important that the project should be kept within bounds, for otherwise the whole enterprise will become altogether too daunting and will grind to a halt. The enquiry should therefore be concerned with limited objectives, for it is vital that the group should feel that they are competent at least to make a contribution to the problems with which they confront themselves.

ACTION AND REVIEW

It is important that the group should see the purpose of the main enquiry as an examination of the possibility of their taking some action. The enquiry should not be seen as a statistical enquiry, but as an assessment of need and of the group's most appropriate contribution.

The plan of action that ensues should be capable of accomplishment well within the time-span that the young people concerned are likely to be able to sustain. A short and limited piece of action—even a single occasion—will be of far more benefit than a more ambitious scheme that begins to run down before it is completed. In any case, the initial action may be a step in what becomes a much larger programme.

As soon as some action has been completed, the plan of action should be subjected to review. Was the assessment of the need correct, or does the direction of the action need to be changed? How were the efforts of the young people received, and what kind of rapport did they establish with the people whom they met? What kind of experience was it for them? Did they meet any unsuspected difficulties, and was the preparation appropriate? Both the success of the action and the value of the experience to the young people will be influenced by the quality of the review sessions. Action and review should alternate throughout the project.

We shall need to raise enough enthusiasm to ensure that some action does take place, and this must be done afresh at every stage. The first steps, including the incentive to embark on the preliminary enquiry, will have grown out of the group's discussion and internal feelings. The preliminary enquiry will have added enough impetus for the youngsters to want to take the project further, and as the main enquiry gets under way their personal discovery of need is likely to be more persuasive than any exhortation from us. Whilst the action is on hand they will need to consider the real meaning of what they are doing, and the way that they are expressing their responsibility to the people whom they are helping.

It is astonishing how persuasive people find their own discoveries. Action research is allied to heuristic education, an ancient form of learning through leading the student to his own discoveries, which feeds curiosity and adds zest to learning. It is a vital approach to attitude change. We seem capable of protecting our established attitudes from anything that we are told, but find it difficult to withstand the force of our own discoveries and experience. Of course, if we hold attitudes that are shared with the people around us, we may still avoid change if it is likely to bring us into conflict with them. But if we can go through this experience and change in the company of a group of people who offer us support, there is a much greater likelihood of our new position becoming consolidated. Action research can be a valuable tool when working with any people whose attitudes may impede their growth or adjustment, and this may apply as much to the training of teachers, social workers and youth workers as it does, for example, to the treatment of delinquents.

If we have in our group members who feel unwanted, uncared for or unloved, who have low self-esteem, who lack social skills, or have difficulty in meeting strangers, who have strong anti-authority feelings, whose compassion is unstirred, who are apathetic or bored, whose attitudes lead to anti-social activities, who are inarticulate about their own feelings, who are well-integrated but bounding with untapped potential for kindness and community leadership, then any of these and many more besides may be touched by a carefully developed piece of action research.

It is always tempting to seize upon the first topic offered by the group as a likely focus for action research. For example, a violent gang complained about the lack of facilities for entertainment and relaxation in their district, which was seen by the worker as a topic that could lead neatly into action research. The youngsters gained a good deal from the programme that ensued, including the status of being consulted by some of the elders of their borough, but the worker, in his final report, regretted that he had seized so avidly on the first opening offered to him. He felt that action research that led more centrally into their violent behaviour would have been even more profitable.

The preparation of enquiries

It will be evident to the reader that we make frequent use of forms of enquiry as a method of work, not only in action research, but also in more general ways to engage young people in diagnosis, discussion and action. The worker will need to develop skill in formulating enquiries, and equally in involving young people in sharing this experience. In this way they are more likely to derive a sense of partnership and achievement, and to use the forms of enquiry more intelligently and sensitively.

If we enunciate a problem to ourselves we may, by doing so, already have moved along the path to solving it. When faced by a new situation we may well ask ourselves: 'What is the basic problem here?', or 'What are we hoping that the young people will achieve through this experience?' With this question answered we are ready to establish the broad headings of our enquiry. For example, following the illustration of a project based on loneliness, we may decide that the main headings for our enquiry are:

Introduction to the general area of enquiry.

The level of friendliness of the neighbourhood and the respondent's personal situation.

Evidence of loneliness known to the respondent.

Personal feelings of loneliness.

Whether help is needed.

The scope for any contribution by young people.

Having sketched out the main headings, we are ready to express these ideas in actual questions. We shall be seeking a conversation with the respondent rather than brief answers to direct questions, so we shall try to include a number of open questions. There may be related areas of concern that have not occurred to us, and it is important that the respondent should feel free to contribute ideas that are uppermost in his mind. Thus our actual questions might be something like the following:

How long have you lived in this neighbourhood?

Do you know many of your neighbours?

How would you describe the neighbourhood—for example, how friendly is it?

Would it be possible for someone to be lonely here?

Are certain people more likely to be lonely than others—for example, old people, or young mothers?

Do you know of anyone who might be lonely?

Have you ever been lonely yourself?

Can you think of anyone who might be glad of help or a visit?

Could you suggest any ways in which young people might be able to help?

The worker who wishes a group of young people, or adults for that matter, to plan their own enquiry will be wise to have done some careful preparation himself. Personally I always commit myself to a feasibility study so that I may consider what such an enquiry might look like. It is not that I wish to pre-empt the inventiveness of the group, and in the event the final form may be very different from my feasibility exercise. But I find that I am very much better prepared with prompts and probes if I have done my homework in this way.

It is possible to lead a group very quickly and economically into the preparation of an enquiry. Try using working parties of two or three people each.[1] First settle objectives, and then go for the general headings. Within a few minutes each group will be able to suggest at least one heading, and you may already have a composite framework for the enquiry. Having settled the main headings, you are then ready to allocate each working party a heading of their choice, so that they can express the ideas in actual questions. Once again only a very few minutes may be required for this to be accomplished, and a representative group may be asked, possibly in collaboration with you, to finalise the form of enquiry.

Role-play

We usually introduce role-play to the group very early in their experience together. After a momentary hiatus the youngsters normally respond readily and enjoy the experience, and it rapidly becomes part of the accepted pattern of their group activity. The physical movement involved seems to loosen up the situation, stir the imagination and liberate inhibition. Young people may be encouraged to explore what it is like to be in the other person's shoes: for example, what does it feel like to be an old person and to have one of them knock at the door? What response are they likely to meet? Or what is it like to be a newcomer in the district, or to walk into the school or club for the first time?

Role-play may be used in both diagnosis and as part of the on-going experience. We usually lead into it spontaneously, arising out of the immediate situation, not as a set piece as it is sometimes used. By spontaneous I do not mean unpremeditated, for the worker may well have foreseen the contribution that it could make, and be waiting for the cue to introduce it.

---

[1] For further suggestions about procedures, see *Socratic group discussion*, page 156.

It may arise out of discussion as well as contribute to it. Often we resort to role-play in order to illuminate behaviour or a situation being described; it will be punctuated by discussion as it proceeds, and will inform the discussion that ensues. As we use it, it is certainly not a theatrical performance. In fact, it may amount only to a little shuffling movement, but it may be enough to have everyone sitting on the edge of his seat, wholly participating in the exploration.

Role-play may help individuals or the group to prepare, for example, for the reception of strangers, for a dialogue with people from outside the group, for meeting people in authority, for undertaking interviews, or, with particularly insecure youngsters, for rehearsing whatever is the next little step forward. In this way those concerned will already have been helped to acclimatise themselves to the new experiences even before the event, and may be able to take a rather bigger step as a result of the prior preparation. The reception of a visitor by the group can be built up into a significant experience. Or a group of youngsters, who are concerned with enriching their communication with their parents through action research, may rehearse their approach to a dialogue with them. Role-play may also be used to explore the group members' own feelings.

Role-play may have an exceptionally important part to play in changing unhelpful attitudes or group norms. It can quickly bring to the surface differences of opinion amongst a group of youngsters who all seem to be accepting the norms of the group with the same willingness. This is illustrated by a group who enacted the exploit of one of their number who stole a purse from the bag of a rather feeble old lady. Several of them soon began to express doubts about the event that a few minutes before had been seen as a 'good giggle'. We do not see role-play as something special, for which we might bring in a specialist: it is part of the essential equipment of the group worker, and needs to flow in and out of the events as they occur.

Socio-drama

The distinction between role-play and socio-drama is hazy, but worth making. Straightforward role-play is more concerned with investigating or practising a part that may have been or is about to be played by a member of the group; socio-drama is concerned with the examination of more complex social situations. When concerned with the interrelationships between the members of the group it can add impetus to their exploration, and can cause a rapid increase of supportiveness in the group. It is often used to investigate the relationships of members of the group with people outside the group.

Pauline was seen as a hanger-on, as she was always on the fringe of this group of girls, and never seemed to be able to get on with anyone. They role-played what happened between them and Pauline in the club situation. The worker asked what happened at school, and in the street, and the group role-played these situations as well.

The group soon revealed to themselves that they continually submitted Pauline to rebuffs and ridicule. Scenes were re-enacted to see just what it was that caused them to reject Pauline, and what it must have been like for her. There were pauses as they discussed Pauline's unenviable position and a tentative suggestion was made that Pauline might be invited to join the group again (she had attended a meeting before), and the role-play moved into how she should be invited, and how she might be received on her arrival. Should they involve her in a similar piece of role-play?

Some seemingly simple social situations are in fact very complex.

There is some bullying in the fourth year lower ability group at school, which through socio-drama quickly reveals itself as quite serious scapegoating of a boy named Fred. How are we as a group to cope with this? Role-play reveals that the staff of the school are even less able to control it than the group itself. But here is a very important revelation: it is not just that Fred is bullied—he seems to go out of his way to provoke such treatment. This seems to be the way in which he gets himself noticed. Fred has no real friends, and his parents keep him indoors rather a lot.

By this time the whole group is caught up in the problem at a new level of creative thinking and feeling, anxious to help. Socio-drama has helped them examine a real situation that surrounds them, and in particular the boy in question.

The scene changes from Fred and the bullies to the three girls who are disgusted by what they see and approach two members of staff. We see a rather helpless, indeterminate discussion in the staff room. We follow Fred home, where his brother sees bruises on his body and reports this to his parents. The action of the parents is faltering and it is clear that they will not do anything about it.

Socio-drama usually requires fairly vigorous production. For example, each participant will be encouraged by the worker to warm into his part:

'Now, are you really feeling like Harry? How long have you been in the district—just a week? Have you moved house? And left all your friends behind? What about your Dad, is he in a new job? And your Mother, without her old friends—is she a bit lost?

'Right then, this is your first day at school . . .'

Further intervention may be required within moments, particularly at the commencement of an episode:

'Now, hold it. Are you really in Harry's shoes? Are you *feeling* like Harry?' (And then, to the bystanders.) 'Is this the way Harry would walk in? Are you feeling with Harry at this moment?'

The statement that the production should be vigorous should not be misunderstood. I am not wishing to suggest that the worker should instruct everybody how to play their parts, but rather that he should help to build up the atmosphere and draw from the youngsters a feeling for their roles. Everybody present should be involved all the time, and the whole group might, as it were, talk their way through the scene being enacted.

'Is this really what Tom would do?'—with suggestions, discussion, even debate involving the whole group and adding momentum to the occasion.

'What happens next? You suggest he goes home? Who will be his Mother? . . . Here is a neighbour coming in—who will be the neighbour? Are you really the neighbour? What kind of person is she? Why has she called?'

The tempo is very important and will depend to a large extent on the direction of the worker. Strangely enough, his interventions—'Shall we do that part again? Now what do you think she would really say to him?'—do not break the continuity, that is, so long as his judgement and timing are sensitive. A phase of action can be repeated several times with the group getting steadily deeper into the spirit of the situation. The timing of the changes from scene to scene is also important. It is wise to cut a scene as soon as the major points seem to have been made and before statements become unnecessarily repetitive. It can be done rather like takes for a film: 'Cut! What happens next?'

This kind of occasion can touch strongly and personally every member of a large group. In a social setting of any complexity a lot of people may be involved in actually taking parts—as many as twenty or more in a large group—and the rest of the company will feel involved if they take part in a running discussion about what is or should be happening. Although the scene is in no way scripted, some preparation on the part of the worker is possible if the scene to be enacted can be foreseen as arising from the events that have preceded it.

Social documentary

Groups who have become accustomed to, and enjoy, socio-drama, sometimes very profitably move on to social documentary. Its purpose is to portray a real social situation to an audience. We use it in the main to enable a group to portray something about their own life or situation to a small, participant audience.

Although social documentary may grow out of socio-drama, its purpose is rather different. It should remain spontaneous, but the performance has to be arranged in advance and rehearsed, and therefore passes beyond the usual exploratory exercise. The new element is 'inviting' members of the audience to assume the roles of the significant people who surround the group. For example, a violent group may portray their violence, and need, as auxilliary characters, their victims, their parents, possibly their teachers, the police and probably the personnel of the court. The audience, and particularly the participants from the audience, are necessarily involved in a running discussion about what is going on. The actual performance will be directed mainly by the youngsters themselves; if they have become fairly sophisticated in socio-drama, the role of the worker will be one of support and quiet encouragement, though his help may be needed to enlist the 'volunteers' from the audience. Being involved in this way may be a very sharp experience for an audience, but after a little tittering they usually accept the inevitable with good grace and fall in with the general spirit of the occasion and of what is being depicted. It can be just as much an experience for them as for the youngsters, and as a technique, social documentary has some potential for community action and change.

When we began using these techniques (and they developed because one group spontaneously began what was actually a form of social documentary) we feared that it might become an occasion for bravado on the part of, for example, an anti-social group. But our fears have proved groundless. The experience usually causes the youngsters to look at themselves with great objectivity, and, in the dialogue with the audience that follows the role-play, they have usually described their position with great insight. It can also be a most informative occasion for the audience. If they are people who are concerned with the kind of youngsters involved—in the case of violent boys, some teachers, youth workers, police and magistrates—some creative contacts may be made which may continue as an extended dialogue.

Psycho-drama

Psycho-drama was developed by Moreno for the treatment of mental patients.[1] He had a special theatre for the purpose, and a number of trained workers who took the roles of some of the other people in the life of the patient. We use it in a modified form to help youngsters to explore the way they behave to the people around them with whom they have emotional ties, and more particularly their relationships with specific other people, and their feelings and attitudes towards these people.

Other members of the group will stand in to take the part of mother, father, brothers, sisters, neighbours, friends, teachers, employer, or whoever is important to a certain set of feelings; the subject's own role is usually taken by one of his colleagues, although it is possible for him to play this himself. The subject directs the scene with the help and encouragement of the worker. As the scene to be enacted, the youngster may choose yesterday's supper-time, or a scolding when he was young, or a recent break with friends, or any other scene appropriate to the feelings

---

[1] Moreno, J. (1964) *Psycho-drama*. New York: Beacon House.

that are uppermost. He will inform each actor how he should play his role: 'Is that how it went?', the worker may say. 'No, not quite. He was really mad with me.'

As the play proceeds the youngster may identify strong feelings that well up in him, and he will very rapidly be seeing his situation with a new objectivity. Many youngsters have told us, within minutes of the scene being started, that they were already beginning to understand the attitudes of other people in the situation: 'I didn't realise that I was such an obstinate . . .'

It is important that a group moving into psycho-drama should have begun to have identified and empathised with the problem, because some patience may be required to elucidate the feelings that are being faced. For example, the person that they may most wish to help may be hesitant, reserved, or inhibited, and it may take time for the situation to be developed. The group must be prepared for patient investigation rather than events of immediate entertainment and appeal.

The worker will wish to plan his strategy with this in mind. He may decide not to approach at once the deeper and more urgent problems in the group, but rather to work with those who can take the situation in their stride and help build the expertise of the group in exploring situations in this way. Groups may also try an interesting and sometimes amusing variant of psycho-drama, in which the subject plays both his own and the respondent's part, physically moving from seat to seat, or from one position to another in order to do so.

Leading into introspective discussion

The worker's ability to lead his groups into introspective discussion depends ultimately on his sensitivity to the emotional undertone of what is taking place, and on his ability to seize upon events as they occur. Later in this chapter, I shall be describing this part of his function as his tutorial role. But the potential for personal and introspective discussion is deeply affected by the experiences of the group, and it is possible to think in terms of strategies that are likely to lead to exchanges of this kind. Anything that carries an emotional charge, or triggers off strong feeling in individual members which may echo from one person to another, can contribute to the growth of personal discussion.

Action research which brings people face to face with personal need may be of this nature. So equally might be experiences through physical contact, personal interviews, role-play, socio-drama and psycho-drama, and especially a combination of such experiences. A friendship study frequently has this quality.

A number of other techniques will lead to introspective discussion: for example, the worker can develop several agendas for discussion that have this effect. When in our research we have been exploring what were for us new fields of enquiry, we have often sought the collaboration of small groups of young people in helping us to identify our problem. We did this when we were wanting to explore the nature of intimacy and the kind of intimate exchanges that pass between friends. In order to illuminate the topic, we invited small groups to join in a discussion based on an agenda of questions, the first few to warm into the subject and the later questions to explore the topic more deeply. Experienced teachers and youth workers led the discussions. Most of the young people whom we approached enjoyed the experience very much, and were led to self-searching and self-knowledge. The exchanges were so valuable to those involved that a number of the workers concerned incorporated similar techniques in their group work. Since then we have used agendas of this kind as a normal part of our work.

Here is an example of a series of headings that will lead both to introspective exchanges and some thinking about intimacy:

What kind of things make you cheerful?

What kind of things make you sad?

What kind of things are really important to you?

What makes you feel really happy?

What kind of things worry you?

What kind of things make you feel:
   (a) uneasy?
   (b) angry?
   (c) guilty?
   (d) anxious?
   (e) frightened?

Are there things that you cannot discuss with:
   (a) your parents?
   (b) your friends?
   (c) anybody at all?

Do you day-dream about:

(a) doing certain things?

(b) being someone or something?

Are there things about yourself you don't want people to know?

The quality of the discussion will, of course, be greatly influenced by the leadership of the worker. It would be possible for a group to scamper through a programme of this kind, but alternatively a group may return several times to the programme in order to do justice to the issues and feelings raised.

Life-space diagram

A friendship study is a very economical way of leading a group into considering how each one surrounds himself with relationships, and whether he expresses a general style of relationship in so doing. But friendship, however important, is only one of several kinds of relationships. It is possible to extend the exploration of each person's relationships through a life-space diagram.

The mechanics of the exercise are simple. Each person takes a piece of paper, puts ME in the centre of it, and then adds in the other important people in his life at a 'relative' distance from ME. Some concentrate people from the various facets of life (for example, family, friends, schoolmates and workmates) in different sectors, though at varying distances from the centre. Others construct a target diagram with concentric circles indicating the distance in the relationships.

Most people amend their first position as they come to question the closeness of different relationships, and they may find themselves asking entirely new questions about their relationships. We may introduce an additional dimension by inviting them to add people who are near to them because of their importance to them, but whom they would prefer to see at a greater distance. The same kind of diagram may be used to explore authority relationships, or the inevitable relationships involved in a task situation. The teacher or youth worker may find it an informative experience to draw a relationships diagram of himself and the other members of staff.

Most people find this very interesting, and to some it is a severe experience. It is possible that individual people suddenly see themselves in a very isolated position and the worker and group must be ready to support those who need to talk through their position.

Self-description

When dealing with introspective discussion, and the discovery of self through, say, a life-space diagram, we are necessarily in the realm of behaviour characteristics and feelings about oneself. Self-knowledge can very often be a prerequisite to self-help. As personal insight is being increased, we are building up a framework of discussion through which the youngster can become more articulate about himself.

This can all be brought to a point of greater definition through an attempt at self-description, which can be based on the kind of framework that I have included as Appendix 2 (pages 195–201). It is not intended as an exact description of personality, but has been evolved as an aid to self-examination. It can be adapted to a number of different purposes. For example, we have used an amended framework to stimulate teachers and youth workers to think about their professional performance. It is the kind of experience that can be incorporated into a longer-term strategy, often as the culmination of a number of other experiences, and as the beginning of a new phase of action and personal experimentation.

There are tests of personality which we have found useful in certain situations, but it is not possible to deal with these, or with the psychology of personality, within the confines of this book.[1] We need some kinds of tests for the evaluation of our work, but many of the instruments that the worker will find of greatest

---

[1] For several approaches to the psychology of personality and personality tests, see:

Cattell, R. B. (1965) *The Scientific Analysis of Personality*. Harmondsworth: Penguin Books.

Kelly, G. A. (1955) *The Psychology of Personal Constructs*. New York: W. W. Norton.

Bannister, D. and Fransella, F. (1971) *Inquiring Man: The Theory of Personal Constructs*. Harmondsworth: Penguin Books.

Semeonoff, B. (ed.) (1966) *Personality Assessment*. Harmondsworth: Penguin Books.

value serve more as a stimulus to self-awareness and self-help than as exact measures.

The tutorial role

The techniques that we use will inevitably have some effect, but much of the potential of everything that we do will depend upon the more subtle intervention by the group worker in the face-to-face situation. This is what I have called the worker's tutorial role. The group worker is constantly helping along the discussion in the group, but in this his function is quite different from the usual preconception of the discussion group leader: his job is not so much to get discussion going as to see that certain quite specific benefits are derived from it. This role is probably best likened to that of the group tutor, in which his style of leadership is crucial, as it is in every part of group work. For example, the worker cannot withdraw his leadership, for he is inevitably in a leadership role: he can be an active or inactive leader, but whatever he does he is still leading and has considerable influence. He cannot avoid influencing the direction of discussion—even his silence will do this and sometimes very sharply—and his intervention therefore calls for considerable judgement. Certain lines of conversation may be more helpful than others, and he can be quite formative in which lines of conversation are taken up. All kinds of issues are likely to be raised. Some will be taken up and others dropped, and the worker can influence the direction very economically, sometimes with a single word or gesture, by causing the group to focus on some topics rather than others.

Although it may seem a contradiction in terms, the worker can prepare for an informal discussion by constructing for himself a personal agenda. This will consist not so much of items to be discussed, as matters of some importance in the development of individual members of the group. For example:

> 'Am I right in assuming that both Jim and Rachel have strong feelings about authority? and has Jean as low a self-concept as it seems? . . .'

It is not that the worker is going to wrench the conversation round to what he wants covered, or to squeeze individuals into making confessional statements; it is much more a matter of being aware of the kinds of topics of conversation that will be helpful to each youngster, and when opportunity occurs, seeing that an arena is cleared in front of a particular youngster should he want to move into it. So much of what is written above about the exploration of relationships and introspective discussion will come to nothing unless the worker trains himself in the sensitivity that is required to discern and build upon opportunities to lead into this kind of discussion. In particular, the worker must be able to hear the emotional undertone of what is being said.

The physical conditions in which the group meetings take place are important. There must be some privacy if deeper discussions are to be developed, and the conditions should be warm and comfortable enough to allow the youngsters to spend time sitting and discussing, if this is important to them. The actual placing of the participants for discussion is important, too. Spontaneous groupings are likely to be ragged, and the worker will be well advised to seek some arrangement by which each participant will be able to see all the others—in this respect, a circle has considerable advantages over a square. (The latter is too often accepted as a result of grouping round a table.) In particular, the worker should be able to see the participants.

This already tells us something about the way the worker should be using his eyes. The strength of eye contact as a means of communication has already been mentioned, and in the tutorial situation it has special significance. If the worker engages each speaker in eye contact, it is very likely that he will establish himself as a focus through which all contributions are made. By so engaging a single person who is speaking, he can easily find himself in a dialogue with that person to the exclusion of the rest of the group. Besides, he needs his eyes to spot the signals that other members of the group are putting out.

The use of eyes is also one of the main means of deflecting comments addressed to the worker to the other members of the group. If the speaker cannot meet the eyes of the worker, he will tend to look elsewhere for feedback. Or the worker may deflect the conversation by not replying himself, enquiring of the other members of the group by eyes, gesture or a word. Sometimes we need to mirror a statement to the speaker so that he can consider more deeply his position. This can often be done by echoing a single word, or by asking the speaker to repeat a phrase and holding the attention of the group to what has been said.

The importance of good preparation and of a personal agenda can be seen in the worker's ability to link one statement with another. If we are able to foresee profitable avenues for discussion we will more readily see the potential of what is being said, and how it can be linked with a previous contribution. Patience is often required and the worker will need to develop skill in storing material—recognising its importance to a line of discussion that may soon be followed, but restraining himself from seizing upon it immediately and thus disrupting the present line of discussion. The worker pigeonholes, as it were, the material, until he can use it either by linking with some other statement, or changing the direction of the conversation by referring back to it. If the worker cannot trust his memory, a single written word may serve as an aide-memoire.[1]

Silences can play an important part in the exchanges within a group, and it is important that the worker can tolerate silence. Some workers seem to judge the success of a discussion by whether there are any gaps. The worker should be free from a compulsive need to break a silence, so that he can judge his timing. Quite often a silence will induce an entirely new emotional level in the exchanges, and tolerance to silence may in itself serve as an entry to important introspective discussions.

Many groups learn to tolerate, even value, silences when the members are busy with their own thoughts. It is interesting at times to explore what was within the silence for each member. Some workers suggest to their groups, in preparation for a particular phase of discussion, that each member may wish to make use of a few minutes silence for contemplation.

---

[1] Button, L. (1971) *Discovery and Experience*. London: Oxford University Press. For a more detailed treatment of the skills involved in leading tutorial discussion, see pages 152–5, and for a wider discussion of tutoring, see Chapter 10.

CHAPTER SEVEN

The worker's strategy

Working towards objectives

The worker's broad objectives and general style immediately determine some of his main lines of strategy. For example, if he sees the youngsters' growing self-determination as one of his major objectives, this will inevitably cause him to work in certain ways. If he follows a policy of systematic diagnosis, a recurring, albeit variable, pattern of activity and experience is likely to emerge. But within these broad lines of action, the emphasis of the experience will need to vary very considerably if the work is truly to be addressed to the real, rather than the assumed needs of individual young people.

Objectives should grow out of the diagnosis, but they will probably be objectives that can be reached only in time, by a series of progressive steps. Techniques will need to be used in a fluent way, singly or in combination, as they are seen to contribute to the general movement envisaged. A model of work, such as was suggested in Chapter 5, will ensure that the worker takes advantage of the interlocking and reinforcing nature of the various parts of the experience. And by approaching young people as full partners in the enterprise, he will ensure their steadily increasing self-reliance.

It is unlikely that the needs of any one person can be expressed through a single objective, for personal development is usually many-sided. In any case, problems rarely come singly; a youngster who is in difficulties is usually troubled by a number of things at the same time. Thus, although one need may predominate for a particular youngster, a suitable programme must be addressed also to a number of interlocking personality factors and aspects of development. All this is, of course, complicated by bringing a group of young people together; not only will each have his peculiar needs, but the group as a whole will have its own set of standards, styles of exchanges, and its social controls. How then, it may be asked, is it possible to think in terms of a strategy to meet so complex a situation? First, let us look again at the kind of group with which we wish to work.

What kind of group

It is often suggested that there is an ideal number for a group; for instance, McCullough and Ely[1] suggest that seven is the optimum number. But this must be judged against the setting in which the work is to take place, and these authors were probably writing about individuals who were brought together specifically for group sessions. There may be situations into which specific young people would be invited, or even drafted—as, for example, with delinquents on probation, or in treatment situations —and the young people thus brought together may have no relationships with one another other than in the contrived group situation.

Probably, the greatest potential for group work is in informal situations where this degree of selectivity is not possible. In any case we may wish to work with spontaneous rather than contrived groups. There are often very good reasons for choosing groups already in association with one another rather than unrelated people brought together for treatment, for there are serious limitations to the treatment of young people away from their normal peer situations. The peers who usually surround a young person may have him locked in a fixed role, and there is little point in trying to cope with behaviour that may be dictated largely by the demands of the group of peers around him in a situation isolated from his normal life. The whole group is the proper subject for treatment in this case. Anyone familiar with all-pervasive peer structures, for example in some working-class districts, will readily see the force of this.

If we do decide to approach young people through their natural peer groups, then it becomes a question of how to deal with groups of various sizes, rather than what size the group should be for most effective work. The worker will have to suit

[1] McCullough, M. K. and Ely, P. (1969) *Social Work with Groups*. London: Routledge and Kegan Paul.

his strategy to the situation rather than hope to fit every group to a preconceived formula. Although there are obvious limits to the size of the group that can be engaged in close personal discussion, there are occasions when the worker may decide to accept the limitations imposed by a large group, and for this he may need to use different techniques. For example, by conducting Socratic discussions through very small groups, alternating with open exchanges within the whole group, it is often possible to reach a very personal level of conversation and to create a supportive, though challenging, situation.[1] Our skill in coping with larger groups may be of particular importance in some school situations.

Here is an example of a worker having to evolve a strategy to meet a situation that affected the whole of a large group.

> The worker made contact with the group in their habitual gathering ground outside a fish and chip shop. There were thirty-six boys and girls in the group, whose ages ranged from fifteen to eighteen, almost all of them living within the immediate neighbourhood.
>
> Normative controls had gradually developed that prevented any one person or sub-group from doing anything that the whole of the group could not do together. As a result, the group did little more than just congregate on their normal stamping ground. They could remember the days when several of them could gather in one another's homes to chat and listen to records, but this had come to an end as one home after another had been closed to the hordes that would now descend on any gathering. Within this situation many youngsters could be seen to have quite urgent personal needs for experience of different kinds, but very little personal development was permitted by the existing restrictive conditions.
>
> It was winter-time, which made serious work in the open difficult. The worker discerned some sub-group structures within the larger group, and adopted the strategy of doing some fairly intensive work with two sub-groups who seemed to be both seniors and to form an inner caucus within the

[1] For *Socratic group discussion*, see page 156, and also Button, L. (1971) *Discovery and Experience*. London: Oxford University Press. (Especially pages 120–6.)

total group (but who were its prisoners just as much as any other member of the group). By dint of fairly strong leadership she induced these two sub-groups, one of boys and the other of girls, to meet as separate entities at her flat. At first she met the two sub-groups separately, but after several weeks brought them together. They conducted a study of how the group operated and of their own relationships within their sub-groups. They rapidly became articulate about the quality of the relationships involved, and about the group norms that were so seriously inhibiting the freedom for individual experience.

From the outset, the worker could see the possibility of the sub-groups together acting as a cell of influence in the larger group, but when they contemplated engaging the total group in a wider study, their determination faltered and they became apprehensive and defensive. If the worker had not offered fairly strong leadership at this stage, the whole process of change would probably have stopped and the old habits would have reasserted themselves. The combined sub-groups laid out a programme that had as its focus a conference for the whole group; in the event, the conference occupied most of a single Sunday. They were careful in their preparation, not only for the conference itself but also for the run-up to it, with the result that the possibility of change already existed—indeed, change had already started—before the conference met.

With the help of the worker, the inner circle took the whole group through a study of the group situation by means of Socratic group discussion. They distributed their own number through the small groups involved in discussion, and as a result of their own clarity of insight they were able to lead their colleagues rapidly to the kernel of their problems as a group. However, they could not have carried through the occasion unaided. They were daunted by the presence of their peers, and strong leadership on the part of the worker was required at crucial moments in order to enable them to achieve what they (and by this time the rest of the group also) were hoping would arise from the conference. By the end of the day, the whole company had not only accepted the need for change but had also made plans to ensure that change would take place.

The conference took place just six weeks after the worker first joined the group. At the more personal level, several individual youngsters had shown themselves to be in quite serious difficulties, and the sub-groups had made considerable efforts to help them in their development. The youngsters in the inner circle grew in stature, and were caught by the realisation that there was no need to be prisoners of the situations surrounding them. Having helped one another and the group as a whole, they were quick to see the implications, and began to look around their own neighbourhood community . . .

It is sometimes suggested that it would be better to bring together people with similar needs. For example, there may be much to be gained from learning that other people are in the same difficulties as ourselves, and this is a contributory factor in some therapeutic and supportive groups such as Alcoholics Anonymous. It seems reasonable to suggest that it would be easier to design an experience that went to the heart of needs that are common to all the members of the group. This kind of suggestion should not be accepted too lightly. First, the overt difficulties may look similar, but the underlying causes of behaviour may be very different from one person to another; second, the peer structure and neighbourhood situation may be of overriding importance, demanding that treatment should take place within this setting; and third, there are often also good reasons for having a variety of need and personality in a group. If at certain points (for example, when meeting people) a member of the group is under stress, the other members may gather round that person offering him appropriate experience, support and encouragement.

However, some of the people in greatest need do not belong to any stable group. For example, many youth workers point to people whom they may call 'loners', who possibly come to the club quite regularly but never seem to be in any stable group in the club or elsewhere. Some of them like it this way, but most are far from self-sufficient. What should the worker do? Should he invite a number of such people to come together? Many of them are so hungry for social containment that they might respond almost to any kind of invitation.

There are obvious advantages if any changes that can be

induced can be incorporated into an on-going set of relationships, especially for people whose hold on relationships is likely to be precarious, and neighbourhood peer groups may therefore offer more security to less able youngsters. Often the youngsters without firm relationships are on the fringe of settled groups, and may be kept at bay by them because of their inappropriate behaviour. Sometimes these groups may be a medium through which help can be offered, but before this can happen, the settled members of those groups must have the experience of helping one another and be ready to extend a helping hand to people outside their group.

Social skills and role taking

Our social performance depends, first, upon our sensitivity to other people, and second, upon our skill in the response we make to them. If we are to grow in our sensitivity we may need to have our preconceptions shaken, or even to be brought to the simple realisation that we may not always be right. We tend to project our own feelings on to other people, to imagine that they feel as we are feeling, and it sometimes comes as a shock to learn that another person is feeling quite differently from us about the same situation, or habitually harbours very different feelings from our own. One of the important functions of intimate discussion in small groups is to enable the members to recognise that other people may be feeling quite differently about a common experience, or about life in general. In normal social intercourse we each put on a good front, and we may have spent a lot of time with someone without knowing how he is feeling. We may also extend the youngsters' sensitivity, empathy and freedom of expression through well-prepared personal interviews—both amongst themselves and outside the group— and by including physical contact in the programme.

Inept or stereotyped social response is one of the problems faced by the group worker most frequently. This may express itself as difficulty in making close friendships, or as the assumption of stereotyped roles, and deeper factors concerned with the individual's self-concepts may lie beneath the overt behaviour. Two quite different approaches to this kind of difficulty are often suggested, according to the school of thought to which the writer belongs: either the worker might lead the individual within the group to explore his underlying feelings or inhibitions, or the individual might be encouraged to try to recondition himself to new roles, possibly inside the group at first, and later, with the support of the group, in his relationships outside the group. We have found it profitable to combine these two approaches.

The opportunities for experience in a variety of roles will depend very much on what the group is doing, and putting his finger on the contexts most likely to serve the needs of the people in the group is one of the continuing problems of the group worker. The group must be doing things with a range of personal functions that call for the performance of a range of roles. Meeting a variety of people may be very helpful, especially if the relationship to each person is different—for example, the authority figure, the confidant, the consultant or resource person, the friend in court, the person who represents the opposition. Meeting a range of people and holding them in conversation may be a most significant experience in itself, and the worker will be wise, at an early stage, to build up a panel of visitors who can be relied upon to draw young people into a dialogue.

Sometimes the need for practice in certain roles may itself suggest a context for the group. Sexual and gender roles may be of this kind. A worker in touch with an apparently tough, hard-bitten and sexually experienced group of working-class girls was astonished by their lack of real knowledge about sex. It was as if everything they did was carried on under a cloak of secrecy even from themselves. The great gaps in their knowledge were complicated by their fantasies about conception, pregnancy, contraception and venereal diseases. The many words written about all these in newspapers, and the serious discussions on radio and television, had obviously not reached them; they were probably caught up in the romantic messages of the pop programmes. Similar situations have come to our attention all too frequently.

The worker faced by this kind of problem would approach it in a broad, group work manner. The growing autonomy, self-determination and responsible action of the youngsters would be central to the programme, which would be accelerated by using the kinds of techniques already described. They would learn how to converse with other people, and any specialists involved would be introduced as resource people to be engaged in a dialogue rather than as informants approaching their task didactically. An ability to discuss the topic with peers of the opposite sex might be part of the objectives. Real life situations would be explored through role-play and socio-drama; and the girls might be led, through action research, to study the needs of young married women. It was experience of this kind that so stirred the compassion of one group of girls who met several very lonely young married women, housebound more by their incapacity to reach out to others than by their having young children to care for, and caused them to consider what they could do to help.

Difficulties with relationships

Since much of our personal meaning is drawn from our contacts with other people, it is not surprising that one of the major sources of difficulty in adolescence is in making relationships of various kinds, and within this wider area there are certain relationships that stand out as a source of malaise. Since older adolescents are so dependent upon their peers, difficulties with peer relationships can easily impoverish their lives. There seem to be features that are special to the peer relationship. First, there are qualities within the peer relationship, particularly in the equal and intimate exchanges of friendship, that are unique to it; and second, there seems to be a special skill in making peer relationships that has to be learnt by each one of us. As I have already mentioned, some young people, who can relate to parents quite easily, who can make themselves acceptable to adults in general, who have little difficulty with authority relationships, and who can even relate to their peers on a functional level, may still be in difficulties with closer and more intimate relationships with peers.[1]

Close friendship is largely a matter of letting people into ourselves and many of the difficulties seem to be caused by some impediment in the person concerned, which prevents his letting other people into his innermost self. Many of these impediments might be described as skeletons in the cupboard: it is imperative to the person concerned that nobody else should see these skeletons, with the result that other people must be prevented

[1] See page 8.

from approaching the intimate self. These skeletons may be real or imaginary. They may arise from our feeling ourselves to be of little social worth, which may make us anxious lest other people see us as we feel about ourselves. Or the skeletons may have grown out of actual events in the past: a disreputable family secret or even one's own past history may be enough.

In fact the 'secrets' are often not secret at all, but widely known in the neighbourhood; everyone is nonetheless required to behave as if he were completely ignorant about the matter. One of our workers described a boy, whose father had been in prison, as living a thousand deaths in case he was faced by this skeleton. Everybody in the district knew about the family, but all were caught up in the charade of pretending they did not. A tremendous load was lifted from the boy when his peers revealed that they knew all about it, but their knowledge added to rather than detracted from their valuing the boy.

Not all difficulties in close relationships have this kind of impediment at their roots. There is reason to believe that striking up relationships with one's peers is, in its own right, a social skill that has to be learnt as other social skills are learnt, and anything in the history of the youngster that has deprived him of the opportunity, or the necessity, of learning how to relate to peers at an intimate level can serve as a disadvantage in later life. For example, we have found that a number of the youngsters in difficulty in this way spent their nursery years in isolated situations, and it looks as if the skill and experience gained in early childhood is of particular significance and is not so easily caught up later. Other youngsters in similar difficulties spent their early years in close and somewhat exclusive contact with their parents, like the little boy who, dressed in dungarees, trotted around after his father with a spanner in his hand. This kind of case illustrates how the peer relationship may have a different kind of dimension and discipline from the child–parent relationship, and has to be learnt as an independent skill.

The distinction between the impediment in the personality that may prevent a person from opening himself to certain kinds of contact, and the skill in coping with that kind of contact, brings us to the recognition that social therapy may have two separate elements: first, the removal of the impediment in the person, and second, catching up on the skill that has not been acquired as a result of the impediment. This would suggest that those forms of therapy, conducted in closed situations, depending entirely upon conversation within the group, and upon exorcising inhibitions and other kinds of impediments, may leave out a very important step if they do not also provide opportunities to practise the skill that has not been learnt. Therapists from the behaviourist school would argue that it is sufficient to recondition the person in his reaction to certain situations without deeper psycho-therapy aimed at removing the impediment. Certainly we have often seen individual people overcome difficulties that looked as if they might have quite deep roots, by exposing themselves to new experiences and becoming acclimatised step by step to some social action that previously they found impossible to perform.

Many of the youngsters who have difficulty in striking warm relationships with peers seem to behave with a perversity that inevitably frustrates any forward movement. It is difficult for a youngster to begin to change his characteristic behaviour without first learning how it looks to other people, and why they find it unacceptable. It is really very surprising how hard we find it to see ourselves in action. A supportive situation is a prerequisite to this learning.

The animal game may be played as a variant of introspective discussion. After a period of private and personal conversation in pairs, each person will introduce his partner to the group as an animal, and, of course, he must justify his choice of animal. The description often leads to earnest questioning of the behaviour described. When a youngster is getting to grips with the way others see his behaviour, he may be a very ready partner in the role-play that investigates this further.

Often it is not enough to see the problems in terms of overt behaviour, for the behaviour will be activated by deeper causes.

Ellen had developed a reputation for promiscuity and the staff of the club were anxious both about her future and equally about the influence her behaviour was having on a number of other youngsters around her. Deeper examination revealed that the basic problem was not so much her promiscuity as her difficulty in making warm friendships. She was always on the fringe of any group she approached, and found a sexual relationship a rapid and fairly functional way of gaining some warmth. Her behaviour to other girls, and to boys also except at the level of sexual play, seemed so inept as to make one wonder whether other people's rejection had not become necessary to her.

Approaching a problem of this kind through the medium of a group will demand an arena in which the person concerned can not only work through the feelings within himself that may be prompting his inappropriate behaviour, but can also try new ways of approaching his peers. And since the group as a whole will be conscious of what is taking place, there is a much greater chance of their allowing, indeed encouraging, that person to change, and of their accepting the necessary changes in their own expectancies of him.

Role fixations

Unhelpful role fixations or role stereotypes are seen all too often. The clown is a very frequent example of this, and alongside his entertainment value and tension release he may also perform some very destructive functions. A lot of potentially creative experience is neutralised by the clown in many groups. Although the clowning is obvious, it is not always clear who is initiating it. This may be revealed by a little enquiry, which may also indicate whether the clown's behaviour is peculiar to this group situation or is part of a life style of the individual concerned. Similarly, the scapegoat may first be seen as a boy who is being bullied, but deeper enquiry may reveal that it is the scapegoat who is provoking this reaction, and that it is his characteristic way of offering himself.

These are examples of the more obvious roles. Even the titles 'clown' or 'scapegoat' are misleading, since each person's role is unique. One person plays the clown role differently from the next; in fact, the differences may be so great as to point the danger of using ready labels. At the other end of the scale, some roles are so subtle and unobtrusive as to make them very difficult to identify, and yet it can be said that in a group that meets regularly, with close and settled relationships, each member is playing a distinctive role. The limits of acceptable behaviour within the role may be wide or narrow, and because the role structure is associated with the normative controls in the group, this is a matter of some consequence.

When roles are situational—peculiar to the situation in which they are being observed—it may be enough for the group to become aware of what is happening for the whole situation to change. But quite often the stereotype role we see in the group is symptomatic of the way that the youngster concerned conducts himself in almost every department of life: he finds it difficult to present himself in any other way. This is a behavioural style he has developed in order to attract his share of attention even if that attention is hostile or painful. There is usually also the complicating factor that those around him are similarly fixed in their expectancy of him, which is likely to make it more difficult for him to change should he wish to do so. The approach to a problem of this kind would therefore have to be many-sided.

It is usually fairly easy to lead a group of young people to see that members of the group are behaving in predictable ways, and to an understanding of personal roles as a concept. An enquiry based on the kind of prompts suggested by Group Enquiry IV (Appendix 1d, see pages 192–4) will initiate this, and the theme can be pursued through role-play and socio-drama. Of a difficult group of fourth-form boys it was reported:

> They came into the room very angry about the treatment that Jess had received at the hands of a member of staff, and of the other boys in the class (although not more than a week ago they also had been engaged in a similar persecution of Jess). When they role-played the situation it was revealed that it was not just that Jess was bullied: he seemed to offer himself in this way as his method of gaining attention. They then considered how they could help Jess, and Roger suggested that he should be invited to join their group. They also debated whether an approach might be made to the member of staff concerned.

Moreno argued that it is a lack of spontaneity in the individual that causes him to offer a stereotyped response, whether that response is appropriate to that situation or not. He suggested that it is this same lack of spontaneity that causes difficulties in relationships. Moreno practised what he calls spontaneity training through role-play, in which he would invite the subject into a therapeutic arena, surrounded by trained auxiliaries, to throw himself rapidly from one mood or situation to another, thus acclimatising himself to offering new responses rapidly and

E

flexibly.[1] We have found that someone in a fixed and stereotyped role may need very considerable and deliberate help in making a change.

First, the group must release the person concerned from his expected behaviour if he is to have room for manoeuvre.

> 'Dai told us that not a single lesson went by but that he was reminded of his clown role either by his peers or by the teacher, and usually by both.'

The pressures are often strong, but sometimes far from vicious.

> 'Sammy said his parents were worried about his becoming more serious and quieter. They thought he must be ill and suggested he saw the doctor.'

Sometimes, as a result of the situation that the worker has helped to create, the person concerned moderates his behaviour whilst the group is in session, but this may not carry over into normal daily life.

> 'When we were all together he behaved in a restrained, compassionate and responsible manner, but as soon as the group left our sessions they would all start the usual giggling and his irresponsible behaviour would reassert itself.'

Thus, for the experience within our group to have long-term effect, the action of the group will need to be conscious and agreed, especially in terms of the action regarded as appropriate outside the group sessions.

It is not only that the individual must be released from a restrictive role by his peers: it is quite possible that he slid into the role for some very good personal reasons:

> 'He said that he makes people laugh because he cannot bear to have people laugh at him!' (Quite frequently the basis for a role seems to have been an attempt to ward off the blow.)

And even more important, if this characteristic behaviour has been practised for a long term, the person concerned may not have any other kinds of approaches to offer.

> 'When both the group and Charles saw the kind of role he was playing, the group immediately stopped demanding it of

---

[1] Moreno, J. (1953) *Who Shall Survive*. New York: Beacon House.

him, and Charles, not liking what he saw, was resolved to behave differently. In fact, he seemed to withdraw almost completely, and we heard very little of him for several weeks. He seemed to be having some difficulty in settling upon alternative modes of behaviour.'

The group had released the controls—had removed the negative influences—but had not offered much positive help.

'Ray was astonished that the group should see him as a "creep", and the rest of the group were equally surprised when they realised that he had really not been aware of his own behaviour. It seemed that he needed continual re-assurance. The group considered, with Ray, what help they could offer, and it was agreed that Ray should try taking the lead in some of the things the group did together.'

Many of the situations facing the group worker will involve individuals, sometimes a whole group, in the need for a change in behaviour, but behaviour to some degree expresses attitudes and personality. Personal modification at this level may need a variety of coordinated experiences, and very considerable support from the groups.

The self and others

We find at the roots of so many problems that we face with young people a deep malaise arising from a low sense of personal worth, and from feelings of inadequacy or guilt. The reference above to skeletons in the cupboard, which have to be protected from view, is often about these kinds of feelings. The way in which a person feels about himself is usually called his self-concept. Our self-concepts are laid down early in life and become a central influence on much of our behaviour. They are developed largely from the child's internalising attitudes towards him expressed by the significant people around him. He does not internalise, 'Mummy says I am lazy' (or awkward or messy); he internalises, 'I am lazy.' This basic structure, although it may be modified in later life, is very resistant to change.

We tend always to protect our self-concept even though it is an unhappy one, and we may defend ourselves against anyone who seeks to raise our low self-esteem as we would if he sought to lower a higher one. We even have an early warning system, and our subconscious being will respond to an attack upon our self-concept before we are consciously aware that the attack has been made.[1] The reader may have experienced this in everyday life if he has tried to reassure someone of that person's competence or acceptability; so often every attempt to encourage the person concerned is parried, and seems to have little effect on his level of self-esteem. We seem to be proof against being told about ourselves and something more persuasive than sweet words appears to be necessary. The experience of being treated in certain ways often seems more potent than spoken reassurance, and we are also much more influenced by what we discover than by what we are told. These are the kinds of experiences that can be brought to young people through group work.

Although our self-concepts are resistant to change, there seems little doubt that they can be modified as we go through life, either by the accumulation of experience or as a result of certain formative events. Unfortunately, when our self-concepts are low there is a tendency for life to confirm us in these. For example, many gain confirmation of themselves as failures as a result of their experience at school. This kind of predisposition tends to be self-fulfilling. The surface manifestations may be awkwardness and defensiveness in the approach to peers, difficulty in making friendships, promiscuity, or compensatory and exaggerated behaviour. In the face of authority, such feelings might lead either to rebelliousness or apathy, and in some cases may be contributory to violence and vandalism. When coping with problems of this kind it is not enough to focus on the overt behaviour: the underlying causes should suggest objectives for the work.

Youngsters clearly can grow in stature, sometimes quite quickly. For example, unwilling learners at school, who are seen

[1] The reader will find this topic treated succinctly in:
Rogers, C. (1965) *Client Centred Therapy*. New York: Houghton Mifflin. (Chapter XI.)
See also:
Staines, J. W. (1970) 'The Self-concept in Learning and Teaching'. In Swift, D. F. (ed.) (1970) *Basic Readings in the Sociology of Education*. London: Routledge and Kegan Paul.
Bannister, D. and Fransella, F. (1971) *Inquiring Man: The Theory of Personal Constructs*. Harmondsworth: Penguin Books.

and see themselves as the failures of the school, sometimes respond very quickly when they are involved in a different kind of relationship with members of staff: they can grow rapidly in assurance and in responsible behaviour as they are accepted as having a contribution to make. But this kind of improvement is likely to require a deliberate and vigorous programme of experience that will *demonstrate* their worth, as, for example, their offering helpful contributions to the school following a dialogue with the headmaster.

Anything that encourages the youngster to see himself as a more valued person may be helpful, but there is probably some special effect in seeing himself as of help to those in need. The worker may very profitably take such a group straight into the kind of human situations that draw upon their compassion and prompt them to respond to the need of those worse off than themselves, which may be done through action research that leads the youngsters themselves to uncover the need. The acceptance of their help is an acknowledgement of their worth, which may be supported by their being seen as valued by other people who have significance in their eyes.

Their acceptance by a group of peers may add to their growth and security, but this will need to be on the sound basis of reality and not of make-believe: the individual will need to feel that he is being accepted as he really is. Intimate conversation can make this possible. An expression of feeling, or a confession of inadequacy, which may seem embarrassing to the onlooker, can be a relief to the person concerned: '. . . now I have nothing to hide.' Self-conscious help, such as I have suggested in relation to stereotype roles, is required in this kind of case. Introspective exploration will be helpful, but by itself may not be enough. A coherent plan of action both by the individuals and the group may be needed.

A self-description may be a very good point of departure for this.[1] A clear self-description will give the persons concerned an opportunity to decide explicitly what kind of modifications they would like to see in themselves, and this can form the basis of joint action with their peers. The venture must be inspired by a spirit of realism. Few people can make dramatic changes, and the plan of action is better seen as a series of small steps, with the possibility of review at each stage.

[1] For suitable prompts, see Appendix 2, pages 195–201.

With clear objectives laid out in this way, it is possible for the group to support the individual in a strategy of action. Take, as an example, a shy person who finds it very difficult to meet new people. The group activity will provide numerous opportunities for meeting people on the group's behalf, and the people who would normally do this in their stride must make way for the person who could benefit most from it. Opportunities to engage other people outside the group situation can also be foreseen, using the group for support, for some preparation for the event, and for the assimilation of the experience. This is akin to the practice Kelly described as 'fixed role therapy'.[1]

Threshold of tolerance and acclimatisation

We have been helped in developing our methods by the idea that there may be a threshold of tolerance for someone facing a challenging experience. The youngster may be encouraged consciously to take himself to the threshold of his tolerance in facing what, for him, is a challenging experience, and to accept the support of the group in acclimatising himself to this new level of experience. In this way he may be able to push the threshold further and further forward in successive steps.

This can be seen simply but clearly when young people (or trainee group workers for that matter) face their own timidity. The group will usually quite readily create roles that fit the individual stage of progress, and they may decide that it would be helpful to role-play the situation before, say, a particular youngster receives a visitor on behalf of the group, or conducts his first interviews. In the final stages he may represent the group in a quite exacting dialogue. And during this process another more demanding youngster may be going through the equally severe experience of limiting his own greed for prominence in making way for his colleague. The concept of a threshold of tolerance is also a useful safeguard against an individual being encouraged to overreach himself.

Prior practice through role-play helps to reduce the severity of the experience when it occurs; alternatively, it lifts the threshold, and enables the youngster to face a rather more severe

[1] Bannister, D. and Fransella, F. (1971) *Inquiring Man: The Theory of Personal Constructs*. Harmondsworth: Penguin Books. (Pages 133-4.)

experience than would otherwise have been possible. Role-play can also be used to review the experience and to help with acclimatisation to the new level of experience.

Little movement takes place without stress. The measured verbal exchanges that are the basis for some forms of group work have their place, but by themselves tend to have a slow and limited effect. It is possible for much of the conversation to become safe, or even 'cosy', and for the group to spend a lot of time talking about the expression of feeling rather than actually expressing feeling. It is the actual expression of feeling that is often most beneficial; it may erupt spontaneously and unexpectedly, and may well arise from experience outside the group conversation. It may be verbal, such as a confession of anxiety, guilt, or inadequacy that wells up in the throat and demands expression.

Sometimes a member will explode—shout, or cry. I have heard people, when describing an experience of being in such a group, speak of one of the members 'breaking down', by which they have meant that someone cried. If the members of a group see crying as ridiculous and weak, then this can be a belittling experience for the person concerned, but in a supportive group, crying is usually a valuable release: 'I don't feel I need to hide myself any more; you all know what I am really like inside now.' The major contribution of objective conversation is to increase self-knowledge. When there has been some expression of feeling, including the feelings for one another expressed by members of the group, conversation in the group may help the person concerned to explore the nature of that feeling, and the factors that lie beneath it.

Whilst it may be true that little development may occur without stress, work that is based mainly on problem-solving or crises may also have its limitations in terms of development. There can be an element of competition between problem-solving and developmental work. A crisis may be the manifestation of deeper conditions, and if we concentrate on the crisis we may be diverted from the main issues. We may merely rescue the person, ready for the next crisis. Developmental work can be likened to putting capital into the bank, enabling people to manage their own lives more adequately and cope with their own problems. Coping with a crisis tends to be a circular process, repetitive and all-absorbing. Often there is little choice but to support the individual through a time of pressure, but it is often better to neglect the immediate problem a little in order to lead to a more creative experience. At least we should be trying to use the crisis as a way into deeper issues.

Empathy and compassion

A lack of empathy and compassion is amongst the more serious attributes of many violent and anti-social youngsters. Although it may be less obvious, a similar lack may be seen in youngsters at all levels of attainment and social class. Some of the high flyers, who are destined to occupy positions of leadership in the community, are no more endowed with a warmth and concern for others than some street corner vandals. In a number of cases this seems to be associated with the experience of having been indulged as young children, as if they have learnt to see other people as pawns in their own game of self-gratification.

It may be a lack of empathy and compassion that makes it possible for young people to beat up other people without themselves feeling the hurt that they are inflicting; though some youngsters caught up in this kind of action do not lack compassion, but seem to have a switch mechanism which prevents their being reached by the suffering of their victims. The lack of compassion may be mixed up also with a low sense of social worth, strong feelings about authority, and sometimes a blind resentment against anyone who can be identified as the 'enemy'.

We have not found anti-social youngsters more difficult to contact than other youngsters, in fact quite the reverse. Once again much will depend upon the leadership offered to them, and in the past there has been a tendency for group workers to be hesitant in their approach to such groups. A group of this kind can react to indefinite leadership and enigmatic situations with great destructiveness, and unless the experience of being in an indefinite and uncertain situation is a deliberate part of the treatment and can be contained in a fairly controlled situation, the worker is usually better advised to offer a more active form of leadership.

It is possible to approach a lack of compassion and low self-concepts through action research, especially if its context leads straight into the heart of the difficulties. Workers sometimes find it difficult to spot a context that might both catch the interest of group members and lead to the most helpful experience. At first he may have to cast around for anything that stirs them or even arouses their indignation. In fact, there may be a number of things that do this, and the worker will need to encourage them to pursue the line that seems to have the greatest promise. His early diagnostic work will help him here, especially if he ensures that the young people are partners in this diagnosis. It is often a mistake to seize upon the first thing that is offered—for example, the youngsters' discontent with the facilities for entertainment in their district—when just around the corner there is loneliness, feelings of inadequacy, guilt, or indignation about the way they are treated by their elders.

We have found that quite a large proportion of seemingly anti-social youngsters respond to other people in need. Their response may be instant, both in its rapidity and in the expectation that they should take immediate action. The worker should therefore have checked the possibility of their making a contribution before he leads them to consider it, and prepare a plan for action research. He may need to move fairly rapidly through the pilot enquiry. The keenness may be quickly kindled, but could be fickle or short-lived. He would be wise to foresee the possibility of action that could be accomplished in short, self-contained units.

Authority feelings

Many youngsters have difficulty in coping with strong feelings about authority. This is so common amongst young people of fourteen to sixteen of the lower levels of attainment that a worker, when dealing with this kind of youngster, could reasonably be prepared with suitable ideas that might make a contribution to the solution of this problem. It is often helpful to get youngsters to verbalise their feelings at an early stage, although this can be threatening to any people in authority over them—for example, teachers in school—if they hear about it. The events and relationships of which they complain can be explored through role-play and socio-drama. Statements and complaints may be formulated and objectively examined, and it is possible to reverse roles so that the youngsters become those of whom they complain, and as such must respond to their own representations. Role reversal of this kind is usually a very salutary experience. All too often the youngsters, in their new roles, act even more dramatically than the people of whose behaviour they are complaining.

In this way youngsters quite rapidly become ready for a creative dialogue with the people in authority over them. The objective is not to induce an accepting and conforming attitude in them—in which we would probably fail even if we tried—because there is often quite a lot of justification for their complaints. Rather we would hope that they would come to see their own and other people's attitudes more objectively, and learn to cope with authority figures in ways other than by confused and sometimes violent rebellion.

People in authority may need help and preparation before they play their part in a dialogue. Some will feel threatened by it, and there is a danger that others will so want to mollify the youngsters that they will act completely out of character, which can reduce the value of the exchange. It is important that everybody taking part recognises that some people inevitably have authority vested in them, and must exercise that authority in some way or another. Youngsters will usually readily probe to the person behind the functionary. In school they will want to know how the headmaster feels when he has to punish offenders, and how he sees his job and his objectives on behalf of the pupils; the policeman will be questioned at a similar level, and the youngsters' imagination is usually caught by the very sincere dilemma of the J.P. who may be the very person that several of them met recently in sterner circumstances.

Sometimes seething anger, unhappily only too well justified, is on the point of boiling over into senseless destruction, and the worker may at best be able to convert destructiveness into creative protest. The case to be presented has to be fully investigated and put together, and tested with an objective observer. Tactics must be studied so that change may be effected, for otherwise the youngsters can so easily build up their own opposition. The worker who came upon a group of youngsters hell-bent on smashing up their school had to move fast, especially since urgency and credibility was added by the fact that similar escapades had been successfully perpetrated in the recent past. Conflict with parents, a fairly common occurrence with young people, is often mixed up with feelings about authority, but I will return to this in Chapter 10.

Group controls

Since strong attachment to peer groups is characteristic of older adolescents, it is not surprising that the normative influences bearing on young people through their peer groups can be very strong indeed. I have already described a large group that congregated outside a fish and chip shop and seriously limited the freedom and experience of its individual members. We have come to call this kind of group a 'ball and chain' group, to convey the dramatic way in which the youngsters limit one another's movement, and our research has revealed that this kind of group may be much more common than is generally realised. Greater seriousness may be added to the situation when the group is most influenced by its least mature or most disturbed member.[1] A clown in a group quite often plays a limiting role by neutralising any attempt at serious conversation or activity.

The sanctions supporting the norms of a group may be very subtle and far from vicious, and may even arise out of unconscious consideration for any member who would be challenged by a change in the pattern of life. Unfortunately, by going along with that person they not only limit their own scope for movement, but they are party to depriving him of the very experience he may need for his own development.

It is usually not difficult to induce change in situations of this kind as long as the worker is clear in his diagnosis, especially if he has invited the group to share that diagnosis. If it is based on enquiries such as those suggested in Appendix 1 (pages 186–92), it is likely to open the situation immediately. We are often helped by the fact that there are several levels of acceptance of group controls, for a frank discussion which reveals differences of opinion may immediately loosen up the position.[2] Sometimes the majority of a group may be merely complying with what they think the others expect of them, and when they discover that they are not alone in their reservations the situation will change immediately. This is illustrated by the example quoted on page 92, when a group role-played the exploit of one of their number who had taken a purse from an old woman's bag—with their

[1] Button, L. (1969) *The Harbourgate Group*. Swansea: University College of Swansea, Department of Education.
[2] See pages 56–9.

approbation. It quickly became apparent that the seeds of change were already within the group.

Group controls are near to the heart of many troublesome situations. Apathy often seems to be catching; and vandalism, truancy and violence may well be a way of life that is really alien to some of the youngsters taking part. Rebellious and anti-social youngsters may differ in that some are maladjusted even to the peers around them, whereas others are are only too well adjusted to their peers with whom they share a deviant culture. Sometimes anti-social activity is accepted as a norm in response to the inclinations or maladjustment of one or two members of a group. These members may be seen as in tune with their group, but only because the group accommodates itself to their inadequacy or maladjustment.

This adds delicacy to the task of inducing change. A more inadequate member of the group may be very dependent upon it as a protective cocoon, and several other members of the group may be merely complying with what is expected of them with considerable reservations. It would be relatively easy to expose this situation and to unleash members of the group from some of the unhelpful controls, but in so doing it is possible that those immature members whom the group has been protecting will find themselves bereft of support. The change of normative controls should therefore be part of an integrated programme that has caring and concern for one another as its core and point of departure.

How effective are we?

The change in a person is difficult to measure. We have used personality tests, but are far from satisfied with them as a measure of our work; in the main the evaluation of the changes that have taken place has been subjective. Some of the changes in overt behaviour have been very obvious, for the routine and behaviour of many groups has changed quite dramatically, and in a very short time. Destructive groups have come to take a responsible interest in their own neighbourhood; delinquent groups have offered service to others, and have even counselled 'the law' about the wisest approach to younger children who may be following their own delinquent path. 'Normal' groups of youngsters have extended their horizons, have greatly increased their sensitivity to other people, and some have taken very seriously their own preparation for responsible leadership.

Changes in groups as a whole have been relatively easy to point to, sometimes in only a very short time after the group worker has joined them, but evidence about changes in individual personalities is inevitably more difficult to produce. Indeed, we have to face questions about whether it is really possible, through this kind of work, to achieve changes in basic personality. There is an important distinction to be made between changes in personality—in the basic raw material, as it were—and changes in social skill.

There is no doubt at all that we have seen very considerable gains in the social skills of individual people, and it is encouraging to feel that at least we may be able to help people develop whatever resources they have. Any set of personal qualities can either be used to the full or be allowed to atrophy. Muddled, inarticulate and timid youngsters have learnt how to cope with other people, including strangers, in a variety of situations. Youngsters who have yearned for close friendships have been able to achieve them. Some who were completely dependent, and were inhibiting their own urgent need for experience, have learnt to venture on their own. Others who were always offensive to their peers have coped with fears within themselves and have been able to open themselves to warmer relationships. These and many other changes have been seen, but do they really represent changes in personality, or are they merely changes in social skills?

Reginald completely lacked persistence, and could not concentrate for more than a few minutes at a time. He had a slight speech impediment, and he was seriously scapegoated by the members of this small group as well as by a wider circle of peers. In the early stages of the work he was continuously a disturbing influence. The group met in school twice a week; after only five weeks Reginald was able to concentrate for the whole of an hour-long period, and his speech was flowing much more easily. The group engaged in socio-drama and explored the relationships within the group, and in particular the way in which Reginald was scapegoated. He came to take an easy part in all the discussions.

Whether the very obvious changes in Reginald can be seen as a change in personality is open to question, but whatever it may have been, it was certainly making life considerably easier for him.

At the other end of the scale, some youngsters have continued in their certainty that they were failures, and small groups have managed a Jekyll and Hyde existence—responding to the worker, but playing hell in school. And sometimes the odds have been far too great, and the voluntary and very much part-time contact with the worker has been insufficient to take the youngsters into really different modes of behaviour.

'The last time I met Tom he seemed poised to change his whole mode of life, although he feared that his peers would consider him a coward if he foresook his violent behaviour. And then in the week I was away there was another fracas with the police, and now he is in detention.'

It seems that the persistent group worker must be able to accept his limitations, and to see small gains as ample reward.

CHAPTER EIGHT

Group work in the larger youth organisation

The tradition of large groups

It has been the tradition of British youth work to bring young people together in fairly large numbers, and although the actual organisation may be described in a number of ways—for example, youth club or youth centre—the patterns have basic similarities. Many could be included under the general heading of open youth clubs, open in the sense that there are no conditions of membership that would exclude certain classes of youngsters. These are open also in the sense that only limited demands are made on the members, and their general style is informal. They offer a very different kind of situation from the groups involved in the group work described above, for far from being groups of eight, or ten, or twelve, they consist of eighties, hundreds, two hundreds, or more.

Side by side with this looser kind of organisation there are youth organisations that are much more formally structured, often called 'uniformed' organisations, most of them with a *pro forma* of procedures, programmes, awards and badges. Their leadership tends to be produced from within the organisation, and may have to be licensed by the district officers before they are free to operate as officers of local units. The reader who is caught up in any of these settings may well wonder whether anything of what is written above is relevant to his situation. In this chapter I should like to examine how the concepts of group work described in this book may be applied to the larger organisation.

It is another tradition of British youth work, especially of the open club movement, that youngsters should be brought together in associate groups of their own choosing, and it is through their membership of such groups, as well as of the establishment as a whole, that the youth worker hopes to have his influence. This means that quite inevitably the youth worker responsible for a large organisation is also a group worker, as his main instrument of influence is through groups of various kinds and what these groups do together. These groups may offer similar opportunities for personal experience and are subject to the same kind of forces as those outlined above.

The structure of the large group with which the youth worker is concerned may be very complex indeed. The total group will consist of a network of small groups with relatively unrelated individuals floating within it: there will be close friendship groups, associate groups, and probably activity or task groups. In some places there may be a separateness about these sub-groups, but in other places they may be completely interlocking. Within this setting the youth worker serves as a social architect. He cannot choose whether he would wish to be a social architect: that is quite inevitable, for he will influence the situation by his every move, and by his omissions as much as by his commissions. He can only choose whether to work intuitively or knowingly, whether to be informed or uninformed, and whether or not to be a skilled architect.

The dynamics of larger groups

Although it is not possible to deal thoroughly with the dynamics of large groups within the confines of this book, it is necessary to identify certain factors in order to move this account forward. There are a number of important streams of influence on the individual within the larger establishment. As in the case of small groups acting together, certain experiences reach him through both the corporate and individual events and activities, but an important part of the experience will reach him through his membership of small groups within the larger establishment. These small groups have their own life and momentum in the same way as those that have been considered in preceding chapters of this book.

The total institutional group is an important part of the environment of the small groups within it, and the influences thus bearing on those small groups may be very strong indeed. Youth workers are sometimes concerned with what they call a 'general atmosphere' or 'club spirit', but the influences are likely to go far beyond what is normally implied by these terms. A more exact analysis may bring both greater insight and more room for manoeuvre.

Pattern of interaction

People working in the youth service have tended to set considerable store on the effect of 'association',[1] but in many establishments the question of how association takes place has remained unanswered or even unasked. The actual contact or communication between two people—or *interaction* as it is called in the language of group dynamics—is the basis for the growth of any kind of relationship. No matter how much people may desire to know or become friends with others, unless suitable interaction takes place a relationship cannot grow. On the other hand, if interaction between two people takes place, whether this is welcomed or forced upon them as a condition of their doing something else they want to do, then it will be necessary for them to cope with one another. In coping with one another they form some kind of relationship. I am not suggesting that the relationship will be a friendly or even a pleasant one, but only that some kind of attachment will be inevitable if interaction takes place.

All this may seem obvious enough, and yet it does not seem to be understood by many youth workers—or teachers. They may describe their work in terms of human development and social skills, entertain ambitions to build up a warm and friendly group, and yet seem bent on minimising the points of interaction between their members as a result of the routine they structure into their work. Interaction may be studied and plotted as it takes place, along the lines suggested on pages 32 and 33.

In any study of this kind we must distinguish between the informal interaction that flows naturally from the relationships that already exist, and the interaction that results from the routine, programme, or structure of the organisation. Examine this for yourself. Choose a small area, either in terms of a space or of an activity, and watch closely the pattern of interaction. Who is involved, what takes place between them, how much mobility is there, and how frequently does the personnel change in a

[1] H.M.S.O. (1960) *The Youth Service in England and Wales* (page 52).

particular area? Is it only the members of settled sub-groups who interact with one another, or is there interaction between a number of sub-groups? Is the interaction at a superficial level, or does it persist long enough for depth to grow? And how far is it spontaneous, or is it prompted by the routine or physical conditions of the establishment?

What happens at the entrance or at the reception area, and how is the newcomer received? If there is a coffee bar, what is the pattern of movement, and how does the disposition of furniture affect the way in which people rub shoulders with one another? What interaction is caused by the formal games and the control of games equipment? How is the institution governed? What interaction arises out of consultation and decision-making, and how are decisions communicated? All these and many other facets of the life of the institution will influence the total pattern of interaction, and therefore the growth of relationships. Although we may not have much direct influence over the interaction that flows naturally out of the already established relationships, these may themselves have been influenced quite considerably, or even initiated, by the inescapable interaction structured into the day-to-day life of the institution, and on these we have a very considerable influence.

The levels of companionship described on pages 49 and 52 have considerable relevance to this study. Some young people will join a youth organisation still in need of close friends, but most will join together with their close friends or are already satisfied in this respect, and are more likely to be seeking or wishing to maintain a wider social containment. If the youngster is to widen his circle of relationships, the necessary points of interaction must be there. It may seem reasonable to expect that the youngster should make the running in establishing these contacts, but our research has led us to believe that such confidence on our part might well be misplaced. The availability of other people implies much more than their physical proximity; there may need to be some kind of external impetus to initiate the interaction necessary for the growth of relationships.

Different establishments vary greatly in the degree to which they provide opportunities for widening contacts, and many youth workers seem not to be conscious of their effect on the pattern of interaction in the institution: what happens tends to arise from the worker's personality and intuitive approach rather than from any deliberate action and policy. Most could greatly increase the value of their organisation to its members by taking thought about the patterns of interaction that exist.

Group norms

The group norms that grow up in the institution may be either of considerable benefit or an impediment to the constituent groups and members. They may vary from the implied question, 'What have you come here to do?' to the injunction, 'We don't do anything here, chum, and we spend a lot of time not doing it. So simmer down.' Some club leaders find it very difficult to stir their members into active participation. This could be an expression of the young people's personal indolence, but it is just as likely to be because the normative structure of the organisation demands that they 'hang around'. Similarly in school, the normative controls may vary from group to group, from, 'The school's great, we are with it and all it stands for', to, 'The school stinks. Avoid work and play up the teachers as much as you can.'[1] Few of us are free agents; if we wish to belong to a particular group we must pay the price of conforming to their group norms.

Normative controls may penetrate into very intimate aspects of life. For example, we have discovered that mating patterns may be strongly influenced by group controls, and may also be very different from one youth club to another. In some clubs there is an expectancy held by the members (and often accepted by the youth worker as a natural social process) that couples who are going steady will automatically leave the club. In other places the controls are different; courting couples are quite at home and many remain in membership.[2]

The ability to recognise group norms and to help the group to break free from unhelpful controls is just as much a skill of the institutional group worker as it is of the worker concerned with small groups. Whether we are the victim of group controls or an influencer of them is probably a watershed between well-intentioned effort and professional work. The worker who is able

[1] Hargreaves, D. (1967) *Social Relations in a Secondary School*. London: Routledge and Kegan Paul.

[2] Atteridge, Y. (1965); Parnham, J. (1966); Jordan, J. (1970) Unpublished manuscripts in University College of Swansea, Faculty of Education Library.

to recognise group norms and influence them, for example through appropriate discussion, consultation and action research, has an important contribution to make to the education service as a whole in helping to cope with some of its most persistent problems.

Consultation

Consultation should be a natural tool of the group worker, and for that matter of the teacher or anyone else who must enlist the efforts of other people. By consultation I mean that we will ask those who will be affected by some action to make their suggestions: first, about what course of action should be initiated; and, second, about how it should be accomplished. There is sometimes some confusion about what constitutes genuine consultation, especially when people see it as a cunning method of persuading others to accept their own ideas; consultation cannot be said to have taken place unless the person who is initiating it is open to change. Things can go wrong, too, when the person consulting his followers does not make sure that the problem is clearly identified (and he may find in the process that his own preconceptions of the problem have not been correct), and the room for manoeuvre has not been made clear. This is particularly important in the case of the leader who is appointed by some outside body, and may not abdicate ultimate responsibility. Confusion may arise when consultation and shared responsibility is thought of by the worker as being 'democratic'. Can the appointed leader ever be democratic?

Sometimes the business of engaging young people in responsible action is bedevilled by the violent oscillations of the worker concerned: he is either doing it all himself, or is contracting out and leaving it all to the youngsters. With some workers it looks almost like perversity: 'There you are, I left it all to them and look what a mess they have made of it', and the inevitable inadequacy of the youngsters is used as an excuse to take over the reins again. The necessity of encouraging and training young people to take initiative and responsibility serves as a reminder that group work is not something that is done only when the group is meeting. When individual young people have assumed personal assignments on behalf of the group, they may need help and encouragement in seeing them through. Much 'group work' is therefore done in passing, propping up morale and maintaining the impetus of the whole process.

If young people are to learn the skills of organising things for themselves, the opportunities for doing this must be created. The worker will therefore be watching for any suitable bits of business that will require the group to take decisions, and individual youngsters to invest some effort. He will also wish to ensure that any contribution to the group by a member is acknowledged by the group. In groups that are rather too large for everybody to be involved in each decision and action, it may be necessary to set up *ad hoc* working parties to throw up suggestions or carry through some action, and, with even larger groups, it may be necessary to form some kind of representative body or steering committee. If this does become necessary we shall need to be careful that the committee members are in really close touch with the people whom they represent, are seen to be representing them, and are taking trouble to keep their peers informed and stirred.

Changing norms or attitudes

There is a good deal of interplay between personal attitudes and the demands made upon us, through normative controls, by the people around us. Some attitudes are near to the core of our personality, and may set limits to the pressures that we are prepared to accept from others. But many of our attitudes are caught from the people with whom we are in association. Attitudes may be very resistant to change, either because they are inextricably mixed up with our personality, or because they are continually reinforced by the climate around us, through the norms of groups to which we belong. For this reason, changing group norms or changing the kind of attitudes that are responsive to group pressures may be closely associated.

I have already suggested several ways in which the modification of group norms may be approached—for example, through consultation, role-play, or action research. But there seems to be a basic principle running through all this that is worthy of some attention. It is common experience that if we try to persuade someone that what he is doing or believing is wrong then more often than not we only build up his resistance and his insistence that he is right, as suggested in Figure 6a.

If we are wanting to move someone from a fixed position it seems that we must look for something rather more primary than the actual behaviour in question. Furthermore, just as consultation must be genuine, so in this case the person initiating the exchange must be seen to be open to change as well. To

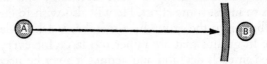

Figure 6a A attempts to persuade B to change his behaviour or practice, but only builds up B's resistance

illustrate from our own professional field: to suggest to someone that his method of teaching or group work is wrong and ours is right can have the quality of putting one person's opinion against another. A confrontation is as likely to arise as a dialogue.

Instead, we could invite the other person to accompany us in a joint study of some of the more primary factors upon which a methodology may be based. For example, what are the needs of young people, how do they behave or learn, and what will face them as they take their place in the community? And what is the nature of the activity in which we should like to engage them? The study will need to move from stage to stage as a problem-solving exercise. As suggested by Figure 6b, it is likely that we shall move through what were previously areas of fixed attitudes hardly conscious of the change that is taking place.

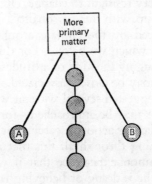

Figure 6b A invites B into a joint study, beginning at a more primary point, and moving through the areas of behaviour or practice

In terms of encouraging responsible action in young people, the case is similar. We can take the more privileged into an understanding of the needs of the less fortunate and the organisation of community life; or the violent, the vandals, or the anti-school brigade into a study of other people's problems and the potential of their own contribution to members of the community whom they could help. The reader will, no doubt, have noticed that this is action research expressed in different terms. The leader of an institution such as a school, club, or department that must face change, will turn naturally to working parties and study groups, but will need to do so with an open mind.

Group cohesion

For most people there is some satisfaction to be derived from attaching themselves to a lively body of people who give them a sense of belonging to something warm and secure. This kind of attachment forms part of our wider social containment, and is an important part of the satisfaction that many young people are seeking when they join a youth organisation. The sense of belonging arises in part from the attachment to the other people in the establishment, but in part also from a commitment to the ethos, the aims and objectives of the organisation.

The aims and objectives with which people may identify we normally call group goals. There is a distinction between personal objectives and group goals: our personal reasons for belonging to an organisation may not be goals held corporately with the other members of the group. We must also distinguish between the objectives of the sponsors of the organisation and the goals held in common with the members of that organisation: the sponsors of a youth organisation may have purposes concerned with the education and social training of the members that could not be further from the minds of the young people themselves. Objectives do not become group goals unless they are shared corporately by the members of the group.

Smaller groups within a larger establishment may have goals of their own, and the goals of sub-groups may be contributory to the goals of the whole group, or may be in conflict with them. This can quite easily occur in a youth club where the interests of a well-organised sub-group—for example, a football team—run counter to the wider interests of the organisation as a whole. We may also distinguish between short-term goals and long-term goals, and consider whether the short-term goals are contributory to long-term goals.

The commitment by the members to a group as a result of their accepting the group's goals can be a very strong force. For example, people may belong to and identify strongly with religious or political bodies without liking or even knowing most of the other people in that organisation. All over the world people are laying down their lives for ideals that represent the goals of the groups to which they belong.

In the uniformed organisations there are usually sets of objectives with which young people may be asked to identify as part of their initiation, although in practice the real meaning of all this to the members may be unclear. But in open clubs there are often no overt goals shared by the members, the leaders and the sponsors. In some cases this is as a result of the deliberate policy of making no demands on the young people who visit the centre, but in most it occurs because the whole matter has not received any attention. In the case of organisations that deliberately make no demands, one is bound to ask whether they do not, by doing so, seriously lessen the value of the organisation to the youngsters who use it. The implications may include the hidden suggestion that the young people are not important enough to have their commitment demanded. One is bound to question how much personal significance the youngsters will gain from their membership of an organisation that makes few demands of them.

Some of the youth workers who would welcome the growth of cohesion in their clubs are doing little better, and, by omitting to induce the establishment and acceptance of group goals, they are throwing away a major unifying influence. It is not difficult to work out acceptable group goals in consultation with the members. Most groups of youngsters setting up their own organisation would be likely at the outset to enunciate, however hazily, the aims and objects of the venture, and it may be the interposition of the appointed leader that suspends this natural tendency.

It is not enough to establish goals once and for all; generations of youngsters come and go very quickly, and each new generation must be given the opportunity to identify with the goals, or, more correctly, to re-establish the goals. This lack of continuity may be seen in practice when a group of young people have developed a great sense of loyalty in the course of constructing or decorating their premises, for it can be very disconcerting when the next generation of young people, who had no stake in the enterprise, show little respect for the condition of the premises. The effect of the presence or absence of clearly defined goals has been seen also in the building of a number of community centres. The actual establishment and building of the centre may have drawn a great community effort, which fell away completely when the immediate objective of building a centre was achieved and was not followed by any similarly clear objectives.

The satisfaction of belonging to a group will also be influenced by the status of the group, the reflected glory (or odour) that it confers upon the members. This is a kind of halo effect. Some national and local groups have this effect and it is regarded almost as an honour to belong to them. Outside benefits conferred in this way by membership of a group add to its attractiveness and cohesiveness. The same effect might work either way in youth clubs, or in specific classes in school. Clubs that are highly regarded in their own vicinity will be more attractive to their members, whereas a club with a bad reputation will have the opposite effect, that of detracting from the social stature of the young person who joins it. It is possible to discern a rapid growth in the cohesiveness, for example, of a lower ability form in school when it is accorded some status in the eyes of, say, the headmaster, or the school as a whole. Part of our strategy may be to lead the youngsters to the kind of contribution that will earn this regard, in order to enable them to be more generous and helpful to one another.

The needs of the individual member

It has been part of the tradition of British youth work to offer opportunities for young people to follow a variety of activities, and many of them have gained, as a result of this, some skills, versatility, a sense of achievement, and incidentally companionship and significance. There has recently been a tendency for the provision of activities to become less fashionable, and for a much greater emphasis to be placed on providing opportunities for young people to come together in associate groups of their own choosing. It is not obvious that young people have gained from this shift of emphasis, for only too often it has meant that foci for helpful interaction have become fewer and somewhat limited in character. In some cases, the worker's single-mindedness has been replaced by lack of purpose and movement. The business of addressing ourselves to the personal needs of individual young people may require a much more deliberate and intensive approach than many youth workers have adopted in the past.

In the study mentioned on page 48 of a cross-section of young people aged seventeen who had left school at the age of fifteen, it was noticeable that most of them had been members of youth organisations at some time during that period, particularly at the younger age. Some of them had enjoyed their membership, but for most it was a passing event of little moment. Most of those in greatest need had been in membership of a youth organisation, but in none of those cases had the experience in a youth group been relevant to their most pressing needs. This was, of course, a small sample drawn from a limited area, but judging from wider experience and from the studies of youth workers following in-service courses in various parts of the country, I would conjecture that the kind of situation I have described would be fairly widespread. The boy who is ever-greedy for reassurance is going to need more than an opportunity to use a table tennis bat to help him to reduce the tensions of life, and the girl who always raises the hackles of her peers is not going to 'get over it' merely by being offered space where she can meet 'associates of her own choosing'.

These are more obvious cases, the part of the iceberg that we can see: there is reason to believe that a lot more remains under the surface. Closer study may reveal, as it did in the case of the Harbourgate group,[1] that youngsters in a seemingly normal and happy friendship group had one another on a ball and chain, limiting each other's experience as a result of the group norms that had grown up. The club leader who carried out the Harbourgate study faced the fact that all this had been going on under his daily observation without his recognising the full significance of the relationships involved. Indeed, his concern for the young people and the very existence of the club may have contributed

[1] Button, L. (1970) *The Harbourgate Group*. Swansea: University College of Swansea, Department of Education.

to the prolongation of a situation that was a hindrance rather than a help to their development. Urgency is added to all this by the fact that he was able quite rapidly to make a new and creative contribution to this group as soon as the situation had been more fully diagnosed.

The job of the youth worker is not only, or even primarily, to serve young people who need remedial treatment; he is responsible for a much wider service, offering opportunities to a range of young people to develop their own potentials. But if young people are to be given real opportunities for personal development, they will need to be caught up in the kind of experience that is likely to extend them. The time that many of them spend in their clubs can be desultory, repetitive in content, boring and stilting rather than extending. Altogether, it may represent a suspension of movement rather than a time of personal development. We are not likely to be able to offer young people the opportunities they require unless we can considerably intensify their experience beyond what can be provided by the large and looser organisation. In order to introduce this element of greater intensity we shall need to work through small groups within the larger institution.

It is often suggested that young people want just what is taking place in their clubs, that the situation is, in fact, of their own making. It is more likely that they are conforming to the general expectancies attached to the open club situation. There are difficulties in breaking through the normative controls when first introducing more intensive group work into open youth clubs, but our experience has been that there are many more youngsters ready to respond than there are skilled group workers to take on the work.

Working through small groups

'But,' the hard-pressed youth worker may say, 'how am I to work more intensively with small groups when I have to cope with so large a membership?' This is a question that may very reasonably be addressed to a number of the sponsors of open youth clubs who are making unrealistic demands on their workers. If the sponsors of youth organisations are really concerned with social education, then they must satisfy themselves that the units that they establish are conceived in a way that makes creative work possible. But many of the youth workers who have protested in this way have had at their disposal a number of assistant staff, who have not been used effectively.

An essential part of deploying staff is also to train them, which leads to a number of pertinent questions. For example, how does the worker-in-charge brief members of staff for each session's work? What is his routine for allocating specific and general duties, and how are the instructions conveyed? What kind of support does he give them in their efforts to improve their expertise? Has he evolved for this a series of steps by which the assistant worker may learn his job? Has he made himself the master of the techniques that he would like to see his staff employ? The worker-in-charge really occupies the role of group worker in relation to his staff. It is unlikely that a club will be sufficiently well staffed for every youngster to be reached through work in small groups, and neither would it be desirable or necessary that this should be so. But it would be entirely reasonable to expect that each member of staff should carry a personal case-load of a small group, as well as perform some general duties in the club.

The club situation offers both advantages and disadvantages as a scene for work with small groups. For example, it is an advantage for the worker not to have to give his whole attention to his small group in order to maintain contact with them. In street work the group will represent the sole occupation of the worker during the whole of the occasions that he is in contact with them, whereas in the club the group may be identified as a separate entity for as long as they are with the worker, but may merge with the general membership of the club at other times. Even then they are within the reach of the worker for continued conversations, interviews and general planning.

Some of the disadvantages can be quite serious. There is very often a dearth of suitable accommodation. Again and again we find groups held up for the want of some quiet corner that would give them the privacy required for the development of intimate conversation. The youngsters complain about this just as much as the worker. I have found groups meeting in draughty corridors, in caretakers' stores, or almost sitting on top of one another in the leader's office, into which other people find their way for table tennis balls or to answer the telephone. Unfortunately, some of the greatest difficulties are experienced in new open-plan buildings. Some groups who meet in old Victorian classrooms, sitting on the backs of desks, can be fortunate by comparison. The extreme noise level caused by an amplifier playing records at full blast can be similarly defeating, for the preliminary contact will usually take place in the open area, before the youngsters have been caught sufficiently to demand quiet and privacy. Many workers find that the interviews they conduct at an early stage, before the youngster is prepared to leave the general hubbub, may lead to a later demand for peace and quiet as group discussions are developed.

When working with small groups, the worker's own identity sometimes gets him into trouble. What is he? He is not what is usually seen as a leader because he is busying himself with a small group rather than overseeing a larger area or certain facilities. Neither is he an activity leader, or an instructor. When work with small groups is first introduced into a centre the worker may be behaving as no other worker has ever been seen to behave. Although the youngsters do question his position from time to time (for example, a man working with a group of boys was suspected of being a 'queer') the confusion is usually much more in the mind of the worker. This kind of difficulty rapidly subsides as work with small groups becomes part of the pattern of the establishment.

Perhaps the most serious difficulties are those caused by the prevailing normative controls of the loose-knit open club. In many clubs the group norms say loud and clear that the members are there night after night to sit and look and wait. Participation and persistent effort may be unusual if not forbidden. There is often much random mobility; one worker reported, when he began with his staff to work through small groups, that they had to 'arrest them in flight'. It must be emphasised that the normative controls are part of the character of the particular establishment, and will have arisen, in part, as a result of the form of leadership offered. They are not the result only of the natural inclinations of young people. In some cases the normative controls have come near to defeating the attempts of the worker to encourage a small group to act together, and in this kind of situation it may be necessary for him to initiate some event that takes the group outside the confines of the club and therefore beyond the immediate controls of the group norms operating in the club. Once they have identified themselves as a separate group with a programme and group norms of their own, they usually retain their identity and their willingness to act together when they return to the club situation. For example, a number of groups, as their first event outside the club, have undertaken visits of observation to other clubs in the area.

When we began work with small groups in a club setting we feared that we might dismember the club into a number of little cliques, but we need not have been anxious on this account. Most groups that we touched not only followed their own programmes, but seemed also to identify with the club as a whole and move into a more central position within it. And since some of the first groups that we approached had had until then a reputation for destructiveness, the change in their attitudes to the club was quite dramatic.

Dual objectives

It is possible to approach even more directly a dual contribution to the personal development of young people, and the well-being of the organisation. This can be an answer to the dilemma of the youth worker who sincerely wishes to help young people in a personal way, but feels that he cannot afford to have a member of staff hive off with a small group for more intensive work.

For example, a club was being prevented from reaching many of the young people in its district as a result of an unjustified image as a centre for toughs. A small group of members rapidly and radically transformed this situation. Through action research, they first engaged the concern of the other members of the club, and they then took their enquiry to both young people and adults in the locality. The way that they conducted the interviews was enough in itself to change the image. They rapidly gained new members who, as a result of the conversations that they had had through the enquiry, came to the club expecting to participate in an interesting situation.

Many groups have been engaged in a study of the potential of their own organisation through a programme of meetings, carefully briefed visits of enquiry to other clubs, and a wider programme of action research. The mere fact that action of this kind was already being taken began what it was hoped to achieve. Other groups have been concerned with providing only a programme item, which has been approached in much the same way. The greatest benefit arises when the contribution is a personal one, personal in the sense that it inevitably involves the group in coping with, and contributing to, other people in a personal way.

Personnel

This kind of development can offer help in staffing problems. Groups of youngsters who have had the kind of experience described in this book, particularly of the responsibility for seeing through their own programmes, become capable of shouldering many of the jobs that members of the staff formerly have performed. The potential of self-help is very great. It can be part of the deliberate policy of the group worker to nurture the capacity for leadership and initiative amongst those who have previously been regarded as youngsters of only moderate ability.

In many areas we have hardly begun to explore the reservoir of voluntary help that might be available for face-to-face work with small groups. In the past we may have been even more ham-handed in using volunteers than we were with our own staff. Only too often a volunteer coming into the club has been left unclear about his role, and may have been either frightened by the general maelstrom, or have felt that he was wasting his time because he was not given anything identifiable to do. There must be many warm-hearted men and women who would be prepared to take a personal interest in a small group of youngsters to whom a little human interest could, of itself, make an important contribution.

The volunteer may need to be introduced to a small group with whom the worker-in-charge has already made contact. He will probably need fairly specific suggestions about how he may begin communication with them, and be led step by step to increase his expertise and repertoire of approaches. His assignment will thus be limited, and be expressed in terms of his service to a small group rather than of certain attendances at the institution. Group work of this kind is usually not limited to the club premises. It may not be long before, for example, a small group of girls calls on the lady working with them, first to escort her to the club, and later for informal chats over a cup of coffee. We have had a lot of experience of leading beginners straight into group work, and the speed with which they gain sophistication is often most impressive.

The specialist activity leader or instructor working in the

youth service has traditionally been engaged in working with small groups, but the potential for his undertaking deliberate developmental group work, incidental to his main assignment, has been largely untapped. The potentials here are very considerable; but we have found that a prevailing tradition can also make progress in this direction difficult to achieve. The expectancies of everybody involved in the situation often mitigates against more sensitive work. The manner of the appointment and the briefing of activity specialists is important. For example, some are appointed as 'evening class teachers' and this immediately creates certain expectancies about their role.

We must be careful not to detract from the instructor's ambition to lead the members of his specialist group to an excellence in the skill being taught, but rather we would wish that both the achievement of specialist skill and informal support within the group should reinforce one another. It is usually necessary for the instructor to change his position from that of the teacher who is at the centre of all direction, to the specialist adviser who is stimulating the development of personal and group self-reliance. The process may represent a change from a class to a society or activity club. Many specialist instructors need considerable help in attempting to change their roles and in learning the new skills involved.

A new structure

The introduction of more intensive help to young people through work in small groups may imply a gradual restructuring of the whole institution, and of the way in which the worker-in-charge approaches his job. The professional side of his work may have to assume greater importance, as he comes to spend most of his time inspiring, guiding and supervising the work of assistant staff. He may need to off-load some of the chores that he has carried hitherto, and he will be able to do this only as rapidly as he brings other people, both staff and young people, nearer to the centre of operations. The principles of group work will enter also the relationships of the worker-in-charge with his assistant staff. Although certain ultimate authority will at every stage remain in his hands, he will be working mainly as a leader of a team, concerned for the growth of his staff in skill and personal resource, as well as for the good conduct of the establishment.

There may be certain conflicts inherent in this whole process that the worker-in-charge will need to approach quite deliberately. The running of the establishment as a whole will be a major vehicle through which young people can learn to take responsibility for their own organisation. In this there are fundamental differences between, for example, professional youth work and industrial management. In youth work the target is not a neutral product but the experience brought to the participants for their own development. It is the responsibility of all the staff to see that this occurs, but when the leader-in-charge engages young people in responsible action, including giving them a stake in major policy decisions, the staff may very easily feel themselves by-passed and devalued. If this happens, there is a real danger that some of the staff will feel themselves threatened and may tend to denigrate the efforts of the young people. The worker-in-charge will have to take steps to see that this does not occur, and to make sure that the staff are put into the position where they may take pride in the efforts of the members.

Youth workers in charge of large establishments often debate whether they should themselves undertake any direct work with small groups. It must be clear from what has been written above that the worker-in-charge is going to have his hands very full in training and supervising his helpers and assistant staff, and he will often be involved fairly deeply, even though only at second hand, with some of the more difficult cases. Indeed, in the larger centre there may be a need for a network of supervision through which several senior members of staff will each supervise a number of assistants and volunteers.

There may be certain areas of intensive group work that are more appropriate to the worker-in-charge than to any other member of staff. For example, the worker-in-charge will need to approach his contact with the staff in the style of the group worker. He may also need to take direct responsibility for working with the small group of young lieutenants, the emergent leaders from amongst the members, who represent their peers in contributing to the organisation of the establishment and to decisions about policy. This group is often structured into a formal committee, and it is assumed that they are elected in order to accomplish some efficient organisation. This, of course, should be so, but it is all too easy to overlook the need of these youngsters also for opportunities for widening their experience and for their

F

personal growth. Much of what has been written here about methods of group work may be applied to the worker's contact with this body of youngsters.

In large measure the worker-in-charge is effective by liberating the contributions of other people rather than by what he accomplishes through direct action, and by offering a focus for discussion about policy and for corporate action. It is a role that often requires a vigorous form of leadership. We do not usually draw the potential contribution from others merely by standing aside; at the very minimum we must legitimatise their initiative, and they may need our very active help and encouragement in demonstrating even to themselves their own ability.

CHAPTER NINE

Group work in secondary schools

The school situation

Care for the personal well-being and development of young people has been a strong tradition in British education, sometimes described by terms such as 'character building', and often linked with the general discipline of the school and classroom. Recently, more specific attention has been given to methods of personal support through pastoral systems, especially as schools have become larger.

The concern of the ordinary teacher both in pastoral care and in maintaining discipline is becoming more deliberate and self-conscious, especially as a result of problems arising from the raising of the school leaving age, of the world-wide questioning of how authority should be exercised, and of the success of direct action by ordinary people. Young people in school have become more difficult to 'control'. A self-consciousness has been growing up amongst them about their own rights, and some of them have tested their strength in battles with the establishment. Teachers have had to become more thoughtful about their methods of approaching young people, and it is progressively much more a question of winning their collaboration than of 'controlling' them.

All this has been accentuated by the growing physical maturity of young people, partly as a result of their staying at school longer, but also because of their earlier maturation; it has also been in keeping with changes in general attitudes within the community. However beneficial may have been the liberalising efforts of, say, the National Council for Civil Liberties in proposing a children's charter, the immediate effect of this kind of liberal pressure has been to make it more difficult for some teachers to carry out their work through the approaches to which they are accustomed.

There has been a lot of new thinking about the role of the school in the community. As long ago as the early 1920s Henry Morris wrote[1] about the village college which he was already translating into practice, and since then the idea of the school as a focus for the community has gradually gained ground. This is an approach that may usefully parallel the more direct help that the school may give to the social education of its individual members. The school may be seen, not only as a building that offers facilities to its local community, but also as a living institution that reaches out to stimulate the social development and well-being of that community.

The school is the one agency that is securely and consistently in touch with young people. The youth worker may have the privilege of weeks, months or in a few cases a year or so's contact with young people. But this is entirely in a voluntary setting and in competition with the attractions of the commercial world, and often with the major preoccupation with mating. In un-attached work, maintaining contact with young people who are most in need of help may be in itself a major problem. The same youngsters will be at school for at least eleven years, and the potential of this contact for helping them in their social and personal development is very considerable. Add to this the possibility of the community school serving as an agency for community development, and the potential of the school which reaches parents as well as children becomes very great indeed.

The reality of the existing situation is portrayed by the survey amongst seventeen-year-olds that I have already mentioned.[2] Many of the serious cases of social inadequacy or ineptitude had remained unnoticed at school. For example, a school's comment on one seriously inadequate girl was that she had been 'quiet and cooperative'. Other cases had been approached as educational or discipline problems, and there is little doubt that some of the difficulties had been exacerbated by the response of the school. The purpose of this chapter will be to investigate the potential of the school as a base for developmental group work. I shall also con-

---

[1] Morris, Henry (1924) *The Village College*. Cambridge: Cambridge University Press.

[2] Page 48.

sider briefly the wider dynamics of the school, and the part that the skills of the group worker might play in other facets of school life. What was written in Chapter 8 about the dynamics of larger groups is apposite to the school situation also.

First, I must make it clear what I mean by group work in the school setting. I do not mean teaching through small groups, although the skills of group work may have much to contribute to this form of teaching. Even when the attempt is made to harness the forces of small groups to support the child's learning, this is still not developmental group work.[1] Here I shall be considering the possibility of informal group work untrammelled by the demands of a subject. Indeed, it is the youngster himself who is the 'subject.'

Advantages and disadvantages of the school situation

Many of the attitudes that young people hold towards school are directed in general to everything that takes place in school, which may mean that if we wish to work with those who are unwillingly at school we shall have to overcome their attitudes of apathy or antipathy. In this we shall be concerned not only with their personal attitudes, but also with the very strong group norms that may support those attitudes. Group norms may encourage their non-cooperation, destructiveness, truancy, or general absenteeism.

When we began group work in schools we feared that these general attitudes would be a serious impediment to progress, but we have learnt that it is possible to break through the barriers quite quickly. We have also found that there are compensating advantages. For example, the captive element of school, which we feared might prejudice the work, at least brings the advantage that the young people can be reached at an appointed time; prearranged spots on the timetable ensure a certain continuity. And the less willing pupil may at first tolerate the programme if only as an alternative to normal school work. This is, however, contingent upon the rate of absenteeism, which amongst the older, less willing pupils, can be very serious. I use 'less willing' advisedly. This group does include many of the less able, but effort

[1] Kaye, B. and Rogers, I. (1968) *Group Work in Secondary Schools and the Training of Teachers in its Methods.* London: Oxford University Press.

and ability are not necessarily related and the effect of under-performance may be very serious. Whole forms may be limiting their efforts to a minimum, and spending much more energy in defeating the school than in learning.

Groups of youngsters often gradually reveal their routine to the worker. Typical of this was a lower ability fourth year group who paid the worker what was, for them, the highest compliment of changing their days off so that they could be present for his sessions. They had worked out a complete mythology about the routine of the 'boardman' (the school attendance officer), and about how long they could be absent without attracting his attention. They would break their absences at what they considered to be the critical moment. It was a matter of pride that they had not been in school for more than three days in any week during their last two years at school. There was an elaborate set of group norms affecting not only attendance, but also teacher-baiting and other sorts of mischief, and any member of the form who did not conform to their general standards was considered a very poor fish. The effect of general attitudes and the way that they are supported by group norms has received far too little attention.[1]

However, the nature of the work does bring its own diffi-culties in the school setting. Most activity in school is subject-based, and it is sometimes very difficult for school staff to accept that any work can take place without a subject label to identify it and link it with a body of facts to be learnt and a curriculum to be followed; that the youngsters' personal development should be the 'subject' of the programme does not seem credible to some teachers. Even an entry on the timetable sometimes seems to present difficulty. The need for a recognisable label may mean that it has to be entered under some already accepted subject such as social or general studies.

The difficulty in finding a label may be paralleled by an uncertainty about the identity of the worker or teacher who undertakes the work, an uncertainty that is often as much in the worker as in the people around him. If he is already a teacher in the school, will he be able to fill the two roles without conflict between them? If he is entering the school specifically as a group

---

[1] Hargreaves, D. (1967) *Social Relations in a Secondary School*. London: Routledge and Kegan Paul.

worker—for example, as a youth worker attached to the staff of the school—how will he be seen by the rest of the staff?

The teacher who does some group work is likely to find that the relationship that he is able to strike as a group worker can be very helpful to his normal teaching. This may operate in two ways. The youngsters may come to see him differently, warmly and more personally, and be more prepared to offer him their cooperation in the normal school setting. The teacher, for his part, may develop new approaches to his teaching. Sometimes he will almost unconsciously apply skills that he has learnt through group work to his normal teaching, and in particular to classroom control. Many of our teacher collaborators have volunteered statements about having found themselves more effective teachers, and as a result of the change have certainly found their jobs more enjoyable.

One fundamental difference between the visiting worker and the teacher or worker attached to the school, is in the effect that his work may have on the identification of the youngsters with the school. If the worker is seen to be part of the school, then any attachment that he draws to himself may overflow into a change of attitude to the school in general. This is inclined to be less so with the visiting worker, who is seen to be detached from the school. In fact, it is possible for the youngsters to draw comparisons between their attitudes to the worker and to the school, which can add to their disenchantment with the school.

The worker's leadership in the school setting

When group work is begun in the school setting it almost always necessitates some change in prevailing group norms. It will be necessary to break through unhelpful attitudes to school, and even behaviour that is acceptable to the normal school routine, for example, docility, conformity and dependency, may be as unhelpful to developmental group work among young people as antagonism or apathy. It is usually advisable to initiate the change at the very outset because, if the group worker allows the existing normative controls to be applied to this new situation, he will have the additional task of breaking through this crystallisation of norms before he attempts to induce change.

In moving away from existing procedures, the worker will need to take good care not to lose control of the situation. If his leadership is very different from that normally experienced by the youngsters in that school—in other words, if he does not fulfil the group's expectancies of him as a leader—the young people may become uneasy, anxious and even hostile. They could refuse to accept his leadership, and if disorder resulted he could easily fall foul of other members of staff. In any case, very little can be achieved without order.

This does not mean that the worker must conform to the existing pattern, but he does need to consider his strategy carefully. The tempo of his early work may have to be fairly strong. If the worker hopes to shake the group free from the normal controls exercised by the norms of the group, he may need to cause some temporary disorientation in the group. The setting in which the first meeting takes place may have a very considerable impact, and it may be possible to hold it outside the normal school setting, such as in a youth wing if there is one, or in some room not normally used for teaching purposes. The school library has been used by some groups for their first few meetings. If we have to use a normal classroom there may be possibilities of making changes in the appearance of that room by moving the furniture, changing the direction of vision, arranging the seating so that there is no sense of front or back and therefore no physical area of authority to be occupied by the worker. The vicinity of the blackboard seems to be an area of particular significance in this respect.

It may thus be possible to arrest the attention of the group and cause a temporary hiatus in the normal routine and controls. Much will then depend upon the worker's own behaviour and he may rapidly add to a sense of the situation being different from normal. For example, his first words might be an invitation to join in an experiment (which can be reasonably claimed of any group work situation), and if the content of the immediate programme centres upon the young people themselves, this in itself may represent a dramatic departure from the normal school situation.

In his own leadership the worker may be anxious to demonstrate immediately his intention of avoiding the more didactic approaches that may be common in the school. Some workers seem to interpret this as a need to withdraw any pressure on their part, in order that the youngsters may take over the responsibility. But the withdrawal of active leadership may, in many school situations, be least effective in producing the initiative and self-reliance that the worker is hoping to nurture, for it can easily leave the youngster without direction, and cause a hiatus that gives rise to uncertainty, inactivity and anxiety. It can be argued that sometimes this is the very experience that could be most helpful to the youngsters, and that it should therefore be created quite deliberately. In so doing, the worker will need to be reasonably sure that the situation is supportive enough to absorb the insecurity and even hostility that may ensue.

If the worker wishes young people to examine their own expectancies and behaviour, and to create a very different kind of experience on which this can be based, he can do so without withdrawing from active leadership. He can lead quite vigorously into new kinds of situations and into different kinds of roles. For example, if a group of young people is accustomed to being taught by listening to their teachers and through performing prescribed individual tasks, it will feel very different to them if the worker suggests that they proceed through discussing topics in small groups, and that they, as people, should be the subject of the discussions. He may feed only questions and make it clear that they alone can provide the information about themselves; he may consult them at every stage about the way things should be conducted and even about the questions that should be considered. Similarly, if it is the worker's intention to lead the discussion to the young people's own expectancies and feelings, this can be done directly by asking them to consider what they expected when they entered the room, in what ways the actual situation is different, and how did they feel when confronted with an unexpected situation.

In group work we are privileged in that any expression of feeling, no matter how unpleasant, can form the raw material for discussion and growth. The expression of hostility is a case in point. It is important that the worker should be able to assume an objective position to see expression of hostility less as an attack on him as a person and more as an inevitable by-product of disturbing people by putting them in new and unexpected situations. It is important that underlying hostility should find expression, for it is possible for an accumulation of unexpressed hostility to cause a breakdown of collaboration, and to impede progress and development. The open expression of hostility is so often a moment of great change, when the person concerned is able to break through barriers to cooperation and to face new experiences.

Coping with hostility is one of the skills that the worker must cultivate. He must be able to perceive the hostility rumbling beneath the surface, and be able to offer acceptable avenues for its expression. It is not just a matter of hearing out some expression of hostility: it is much more a question of engaging with the person voicing it, who must feel that the worker is considering what is being said and is being influenced by it. But it is unlikely that he will be helped if he feels that the worker is being pushed over by it.

This is a principle that probably holds true for most leadership situations. Deprived of any outlet, it is possible for the follower to be choked and seriously impeded in his activity by his own unexpressed hostility. In school this may mean that the youngster ceases to learn, and yet many school situations seem to be designed so that hostility may not be overtly expressed.

Socratic group discussion

The teacher or group worker will need to learn a few simple skills for involving people in discussion and group study, especially when coping with rather more than the dozen or so people that can be involved in face-to-face discussion. It is relatively easy to stimulate discussion amongst fairly large groups by breaking them into small groups of three or four people, and posing a series of questions. When a question has been discussed by the small groups for a few minutes, the worker may call for the attention of the whole group so that they may report to one another the salient points that have arisen in the small groups. The exchanges between the small groups will lead quite naturally into the next question, which is fed to the small groups. We call this Socratic group discussion, which in many ways is like programmed learning. An important skill in conducting it is to foresee a series of questions each of which represents a small step forward; the jump between one question and the next must be small enough for the participants to make it on their own initiative.

As the participants gain in boldness, they may suggest that the person leading the discussion has already decided what conclusion should be drawn from the discussion before he has asked the question. It is true that someone experienced in this method of work will be able to judge fairly accurately what is likely to be the outcome of the discussions, and therefore to prearrange a programme of questions. But if it is to be a real dialogue, then everybody concerned, including the person conducting it, must be open to change. It is important that this should be both enunciated and demonstrated by the course of events. Anyone who wishes to conduct a study in this manner must certainly not expect the ball to be returned neatly to his chest each time; he must be ready to reach out for it. It is usually a creative experience for the leader as well as for the other participants, for he is sure to have new ideas presented to him at almost every session. We have found that many of the teachers who have learnt this technique for the purpose of group work are soon carrying it into their normal teaching.[1]

Discussion about ourselves often involves us in certain abstractions, and some groups in school, especially but not exclusively the lower ability groups, need to be warmed up for this kind of exchange. For example, if we are wanting to discuss personal relationships with a middle to lower ability group of school leavers, who have not been accustomed to discussion in the classroom, it is likely that we shall have some difficulty in getting it off the ground. It is unlikely that they will be able to discuss at even a simple level of abstraction and we may have to begin at simple memory recall. For example, the early stages of a programme of discussion about relationships might run like this:

> After a very brief introduction inviting the young people to collaborate in this experience or experiment, we would suggest working in small groups of, say, three or not more than four people. What kind of groups should these be? We could choose: (*a*) to work with our pals, the people we know well and feel at home with; or (*b*) to try working with people we do not know so well. Is there a case for including both boys and girls in the same group? Turn to your neighbour and discuss this for a minute or two. Now, what kind of groups would you like?

[1] For some examples of Socratic group discussion see Button, L. (1971) *Discovery and Experience*. London: Oxford University Press. (Especially pages 36–7 and 120–6.)

It is fairly predictable that members will choose to work with their pals with whom they feel at home. Then why raise the question? First, the idea of other possibilities has been planted, and we intend to return to this later; and, second, they have already been consulted about something and have been party to a decision about the way that the proceedings should be conducted.

Once the small groups are arranged, the meeting might proceed in this way.

> Can we help one another to remember who were the first two people whom we met this morning? Tell the other members of your group. Help one another to remember.

Here is simple memory recall; but if the participants have had little experience of approved talking in class, it may be difficult for them to converse even at this level. It is helpful for the worker to move around quickly in order to prompt the small groups in their discussion. It may require only two or three minutes for this task to be accomplished, and it is a mistake to leave it too long because attention will wander. In any case, the discussion in small groups is not intended to exhaust the topic, but rather to stir ideas that may contribute to the open discussion that follows.

> Raise your heads. No, don't move from your small groups— we shall be back there in a few minutes. Now, who were the first two people you met this morning?

We encourage one group after another to contribute to the open discussion. Many of them will be very timid and it will be impossible to hear them beyond their immediate group. It may be necessary for us to move near to the youngster speaking and to repeat what he says for all to hear. As members become bolder we may be able to place ourselves farther and farther away from where they are speaking, thus encouraging them all the time to speak out more loudly. But we may have to respond to each youngster differently, according to his stage of development. In moving around we shall need to watch our own placing carefully. Whilst we may wish to make ourselves personally available to the youngster who is speaking, we shall also need to make sure that we are symbolically including everyone else in the exchange.

In the beginning the worker may find himself very much the focus for all the exchanges. As the participants become accustomed to the situation, bolder and more skilled—all of which may happen with remarkable rapidity—it may be possible to deflect many of the comments directed at the worker for the response of other people. Thus a dialogue will develop across the group without making use of the worker as an intermediary. However, the central position of the worker also has its advantages: it allows him to intervene, often to suggest matters that appear to have been overlooked by the small groups, to add points of emphasis, to crystallise conclusions, and above all to influence the tone of the occasion.

Perhaps the most important element underlying the success of the enterprise is the general tone, and especially the support that individuals feel when attempting to make their contributions. Central to this is the willingness of the youngsters to listen to one another. We find that many children in school just do not listen to what the other person is saying; they seem only to be centred on the teacher, sometimes vying competitively with one another for his attention. We may need to appeal to their fellow feeling for those who are attempting something which is quite difficult and a little frightening. It is often profitable to make this the topic of a brief discussion in small groups:

> Some people are shy about speaking out in class. How can we help them? Can we discuss this for a moment in our small groups?

The small groups may not offer many suggestions, but the object of the discussions is also to focus on the problem, and we may be able to feed in the idea of the importance of listening to one another. In fact, we may deliberately use the small groups for discussion about any behaviour that needs to be modified or even reinforced. We find that in this way it is possible to ease destructive group norms, and nurture more helpful ones.

The small groups may thus have a range of functions. We discourage them from formalising themselves, in the sense of appointing a chairman or spokesman, but rather lead them into a responsibility for nurturing the growing confidence of each member of the group. The brief discussion seems to have the effect of giving the individual an opportunity to formulate his ideas tentatively and almost to rehearse his statement. He also seems to feel that he has the support of at least his small group in putting forward his ideas.

Although enthusiasm and ease of exchange may develop during the first session, the beginning of the next may be very disappointing. It is sometimes as if each session must have a warming up period. We have found that we can accelerate this by role-play or socio-drama, probably based on a topic that was raised during the previous session. Role-play and socio-drama may play as significant a part in work with large groups as it does with small groups.

To return to the programme already begun, after we have assembled a list of the people whom the members met when they first awoke, we can extend this by discovering other people whom they remember from contacts during, say, the earlier part of the morning. Next we may wish to focus on the *important* people within the list that has been assembled. Some youngsters find even this level of abstraction difficult at first, and we may have to discuss what is meant, for example, by 'important'. We may go on to ask them to describe to one another what happened when they met one of these people this morning, and after a brief report sharpen the question by asking how they *treated* one another when they met.

The purpose of the programme would be to take group members, step by step, into a deeper understanding and examination of their relationships. For example, as the programme progresses we might focus on the differences in the relationship between parents and friends, parents and teachers, teachers and policemen. It will be very easy to bring the discussion to a deeper consideration of friendship. And discussion about friendship will lead naturally to loneliness and the expressions of feelings about loneliness, and without much difficulty the group might be led into action research, giving rise to empathy and compassion, and to some contribution to other people.

Socratic discussion in small groups is an effective way of activating young people, may greatly accelerate the exploration of ideas, and produce an excellent level of participation. In fact, it is possible for everybody to be working all the time, even during the open discussion. The fact that everybody has formulated some ideas means that all are caught up in everything that happens. This type of discussion is also very simple to initiate. Much will be achieved merely by following the kind of mechanics outlined above, but success is also influenced by the performance of the person leading the discussion. His timing is important; often events should be moved forward at a lively pace, but there are times when a pause adds to the depth of contemplation. The whole process should be enjoyable and a little fun will often also deepen the seriousness of the discussion. The worker will need to be sensitive to the feelings of the people concerned as well as to the overt events. He will need to convey warmth and encouragement, so that diffident youngsters may find support for their first attempts to speak out in the open.

Although Socratic discussion is included in a chapter dealing with work in school, it is equally appropriate to many other situations. It is often profitable to break down a group as small as eight or ten people into twos or threes in order to speed up personal participation, the exploration of feelings, or planning the group's programme.

Social diagnosis

The diagnostic procedures already outlined are appropriate to the school situation, although something a little more formal may also be both possible and acceptable, so long as it is handled with sensitivity. Some of the tests may be fitted into the normal classroom situation, and the extra time that may thus be available may mean that the occasion can be rather more relaxed, and the opportunity for experience presented by the tests can be exploited to the full. For example, if personality or self-assessment tests were to be used, they could be a most creative exercise for lesson time.

Though the pupils may readily accept as natural to the school situation that certain tasks must be accomplished, the worker will be anxious that the youngsters should share in decisions about the programme. But once the decision has been taken, it can be a luxury that something appropriate to normal lesson time should be accomplished within the usual timetable. The teacher who is acting as group worker with groups that he also teaches may be able to integrate the two sides of this work with considerable profit to both. Or the worker may enlist the cooperation of other members of staff who may be able to capitalise through, for instance, creative writing, on the interest being raised in the pupils by the project.

Private and intimate conversation between the pupil and the worker is as important in the school situation as elsewhere. There is both value and danger in the existence of good school records. They can help to alert the worker to some of the problems likely to be encountered, but if they were seen as obviating the necessity for, say, interviews about personal background, some vital points for personal contact and conversation could be lost. With the large numbers that may have to be dealt with in the school setting, personal interviews may be a heavy commitment. Usually it is difficult to fit them into the time set aside for group work, for in these periods the whole group must be occupied if the tempo is not to fall. Beyond these periods, any contact can easily encroach on the pupil's other school work as well as on the time of the worker. The worker may need to seize moments that are already broken into by other events, or meet individual young people in breaks, lunch-time, or immediately after school. It is important, from this point of view, that the group worker's role should be understood. He is not at work only when he is timetabled with his group, and his timetable must make allowance for extra-classroom work.

Workers sometimes overcome the difficulty of conducting intimate interviews by using small groups of young people as their own interviewers. When considering the purpose of the exercise, young people often put forward a rationale that would do justice to an experienced group worker. In interviewing one another they may make use of a standard form or something that they have worked out for themselves. The worker can move round to express his interest and to encourage the depth of the enquiry, and he will then be provided with information gathered by the work of the whole group. Although this lacks the personal and private conversation between the individual young person and the worker, it carries something of the same kind of feeling and much besides. Because they have been describing themselves in a situation that includes the worker, the feeling of an intimate conversation seems in many cases to overflow to him. Any limitation is more often in the imagination of the worker, for since he has not been immediately at the other end of the conversation it may be difficult for him to appreciate the feelings flowing towards him. This procedure may also carry a bonus in that each youngster strikes a bond with the person who has interviewed him, and even beyond this one person to the others who have been involved in the same experience. This can accelerate the growth of support in the group.

The experience

The topics used as contexts for group work and the programmes of experience suggested above are appropriate also for the school situation, which in this respect also has some advantages. For example, in school, as a learning situation, it is often more acceptable to young people that some of the programme should be concerned with information. This can enter a study of personal relationships, personal responsibility in the community, sexual knowledge and roles, and a wide range of moral issues. There is a growing volume of resource material to support this kind of programme.[1]

However, it is just as important in school as in any other situation that the acquisition of knowledge and information should be approached mainly through the initiative of young people. For example, 'citizenship' is all too often approached as a body of knowledge about government and organisation, rather than a sense of responsibility that cannot be discharged without our being in possession of certain knowledge. Democracy is essentially an attitude to other people and a mode of approach to communal affairs. It is unlikely to be learnt in a didactic situation, or under authoritarian leadership, the responses to which are more likely to be submission or rebellion.

The school situation also offers excellent opportunities for meeting interesting people, including the head and other members of the school community. In issuing invitations to people from outside the school we have the luxury of being reasonably sure that the youngsters will be there, which we cannot rely upon completely in the non-captive situation. In common with other situations, it is important that the visiting specialist should be seen as a resource person to be held in a dialogue by the young people, rather than as a specialist speaker. Time must therefore be set aside for the preparation of the youngsters for the dialogue.

Young people of even moderate ability will often respond to the opportunity deliberately to train themselves in certain social skills, such as expressing themselves more fluently, first in small

[1] See the list of material at the end of this chapter (page 174).

groups, then in larger groups of peers, and later in groups that may include some strangers. Many are also very keen to learn how to conduct discussions in which they may help one another with encouragement and criticism. They are often also ready to submit themselves to a systematic programme of experience that they see may increase their own powers of leadership and initiative. I would emphasise that it is not merely that they will accept these elements as part of a programme of work; it may be much more positive than that. They may often overtly declare their determination to give themselves to experiences likely to raise their competence in this kind of way.

In the school setting it seems no more difficult than in other circumstances to lead young people into an expression and an examination of their feelings, for example, about authority, parents, and themselves. The last may include their fears and their feelings of guilt and of personal inadequacy. Programmes may also be focussed on the school itself. For example, when helping young people to achieve empathy, compassion, or a feeling of worth by engaging them in service to other people, some of that service may be within the school. Some groups who have become concerned with loneliness have begun considering how they care for one another in their own class, and have evolved a system or routine to make sure that this does not go by default. Groups have examined the position and feelings of first-formers when they joined the school. Several groups, who have become skilled in Socratic group discussion, have helped a teacher to introduce discussion of this kind to younger forms who have had little experience of learning through discussion.

Feelings about school

It seems almost inevitable that when we conduct informal group work in the school setting we shall soon be faced by the expression of strong feelings about school, particularly, but by no means exclusively, amongst less willing pupils. This happens so frequently that the group worker would be wise not to begin work without first considering how he will face these events if they occur. I am not suggesting that this is a disadvantage when working in school but quite the contrary. It can provide us with a creative point of departure, from which we may lead young people to work their way through these feelings, to improve their attitudes to school and their motivation to work, and as a vehicle for launching young people into other aspects of their personal development.

In order to prepare for this kind of situation the group worker or teacher will need to look to his wider containment within the school. Some of his colleagues may be highly critical of him if they come to know that he is listening to criticism of the school. And they may very well see his easy relationships with troublesome youngsters as 'letting down the discipline of the school'. Additional difficulty is added to the situation by the youngsters' tendency to talk in concrete rather than abstract terms. Whereas we may find it acceptable that youngsters should make a plea that their teachers should be more prepared to listen to them or to talk with them at a more personal level, it is more likely that the youngsters will want to complain that when they ask Mr X a question he just shouts at them and so they are afraid to say anything at all in class.

Since the group worker is often invited to work first with the apathetic, rebellious, or anti-social youngsters in school it is likely that this kind of topic will loom large in the early phases of his work. Apathy is often more difficult to cope with than hostility, especially since the same apathy as is shown at school may have invaded other areas of life. Although apathy may in some measure be part of the personality of the individual, it is also an attitude of mind which may be caught from peer groups and neighbourhood groups, or can be induced by the recurring experiences met by the youngsters. Apathy may be a valid and appropriate adjustment to situations that the victim is powerless to change, for it may save him the pain of continuous defeat. It is very often associated with recurring failure and a low sense of social worth. Apathetic groups are sometimes very difficult to stir, and the first signs of success may be when apathy gives way to hostility, indignation, or anger. The school is a likely target for some of this. Some of the apathy to school will arise from the feelings about authority embedded in the youngsters, and may best be dealt with in this way.

The worker and his colleagues

If the worker is to survive in school, the head and other members of staff must share his sense of achievement at the first stirrings of an active grasp of life, even if these are expressed as hostility to the school. It is a regrettable fact that some young people have been hurt by their experiences at school. Some of those who have failed are obvious examples, but the more subtle forms of devaluation often go unrecognised. The distance that has been maintained between the teacher and pupil is felt by many youngsters as being treated as less than a person. Sarcasm and other belittling behaviour by the teacher may bite deep into the self-feelings of the youngster, especially when the teacher unknowingly joins the youngster's peers in thrusting him into an unhelpful role.

Although it is possible for the worker to lead the youngster to some compensatory experience through topics other than school, it seems sometimes as if real restitution can only come from the source of the original hurt. This may mean that a dialogue must be opened between the school as an establishment and the youngsters concerned. In this way they may feel that their grievances are being considered, and that they are being treated in ways that respond to their needs for acceptance and significance. Some workers who, although working in the school, have not been seen by the youngsters as part of the school, have felt that their work has fallen short of what it might have achieved because the youngsters did not see their new experiences as emanating from the school, and therefore as a restitution by the school.

It is important that the worker should not be seen or see himself as working as a separate entity. He should be rubbing shoulders continually with other members of staff, and considering quite deliberately the means by which he can engage other people's interest in what he is trying to do. He can involve certain members of staff in case conferences about particular youngsters, and there is so often at least one member of staff who takes a particular interest in even the difficult youngster. Other members of staff may be pleased to focus some of their normal teaching on the topics being followed by the groups—for example, through English and creative writing. It is especially important that the group worker should convey the order, structure and discipline of his work, but in order to do this adequately, he will need to be well-informed, clear-minded, and articulate about what he is attempting.

Coping with large numbers

One of the difficulties of fitting group work into the school timetable is that the worker may have to accept the usual teaching unit as a basis for group work, and the numbers in the form or set may be greater than he would wish. In some schools arrangements are made for smaller groups of youngsters to meet for pastoral care or social education, but this is by no means universal. The worker must therefore learn how to handle larger numbers, and the more formal element attached to the school situation may be helpful to him in doing so.

More intensive developmental group work usually takes place in groups of no more than twelve to fifteen members, though, as I have already mentioned, we may need to work with a natural group rather than choose the size of a group. As the group gets larger there is a great deal for the worker to keep pace with if he has the ambition to address himself to the specific needs of each person. The exploration of relationships, introspective discussion and the creation of a close supportive climate all become rather different kinds of problem as the size of the group is increased. Although as many as thirty people may feel fully involved in socio-drama, to keep everybody in a group of that size busy and committed to, say, action research, will require very good planning and organisation.

It is possible for exchanges within a large group to become warm, supportive and fairly intimate by using Socratic group discussion, and it may also be possible, in this kind of situation, to deal with personal problems that touch the group as a whole, such as persistent scapegoating. A further possibility is to combine some corporate work with programmes for small groups. For example, a class of, say, thirty pupils can work both as a corporate body and as three groups of about ten people, each group following its own programme.

In leading into this kind of situation the early corporate meetings would be used, first, to gain the willing participation of the group as a whole and the acceptance of personal responsibility for the programme; second, to identify points of common interest and concern and to determine possible courses of action; and third, to invite the young people to form groups of their own choosing centred around the specific topics that interested them most. All this could be achieved in a corporate situation by working through Socratic discussion in small groups. If the emphasis beyond this point is to be on the work of small groups, then the corporate sessions will be used for any revisions of the overall purpose or plan of the project, and for the small groups to inform one another about their experience. But it is equally possible for a whole group to continue with a corporate programme, with each small group contributing to the sessions, or taking responsibility for a particular session.

The major difficulty in all this is for the worker to make himself available to small groups with sufficient privacy and leisure to develop more intimate conversation. This difficulty can be met by careful planning, and particularly by timetabling the steps to be taken by each small group. In approaching this, a firm appreciation of the elements of the work depicted by Figure 5 (see page 75) can be of special value. Let us assume that three groups each have their own programme. Each group will need to take a good deal of the responsibility for its own planning, and it is possible for the worker to help all three groups meeting simultaneously, though separately, in the same room. At the next stage it may be possible for each group to carry through its activities with only the general encouragement and oversight of the worker. This will necessarily be the case when, for example, individual members or sub-sections of the groups are involved in action research or community service. The element that is more likely to need the individual attention of the worker is at the time for taking stock, when each group may be led into more exploratory and intimate exchanges. If the period when each group meets for its stock-taking is planned to coincide with times when the other groups are engaged in action, it is possible for the worker to give some undivided attention to each group in turn.

In working in this way the worker may have to accept a slower rate of development than if he were to give a small group his whole attention, but his influence does reach many more people. The sophistication of the work may suffer in that the worker will not be able to give the same attention to individual detail, but everybody concerned may nonetheless have a very significant experience. The quality of the experience will be influenced considerably by the preparatory programme, which should induce self-reliance both in individual young people and in the small groups, and a sense of supportiveness in the group as a whole. Greater depth will be added to the experiences if the worker can bring the groups to an acceptance of the need to help one another in a personal way, and help them acquire some skill in doing so.

Other aspects of school life

The group worker can help his colleagues in their efforts to maintain contact and gain the identification especially of the pupils of average and below average ability, and of those who spend their last years unwillingly at school. It is vital that all pupils should feel themselves to be partners in their own education, and in achieving this the work of the teacher and of the group worker overlaps. It is second nature to the group worker to foster personal contacts and to put the youngster in a responsible and strong position. In serious cases of widespread antipathy and alienation, a deliberate programme of Socratic group discussion, role-play, role-reversal, and action research may be required.

It should not be thought that problems of this kind are restricted to the lower ability or less tractable pupils: those following more academic programmes may also be involved. Throughout the school there may be under-performance, involving small groups or sometimes even whole forms. This may be as a result of the level of individual motivation, but is as likely to be bound up with attitudes held in common by groups of pupils, or with the pressures of group norms.

The high flyers may need similar help in their personal development. For example, a timid sixth form girl revealed during the very first session of Socratic group discussion that this was the first time she had ever dared to make a contribution to a discussion in class. The more able may also be in need of information, for example, about sex, and may require opportunities to discuss sexual feeling and gender roles.

Pastoral work

In many schools an attempt is made to offer this kind of help and support through a pastoral system. The pastoral unit may be a form, or it may be a special group brought together for this purpose with a member of staff designated as 'tutor' to the group.

In some schools the pastoral unit includes a range of both ages and ability.

The structure of pastoral care has usually received more thought than the actual events that should make up a pastoral occasion. Indeed, in many schools in which a pastoral or counselling session has been added to the timetable, it has proved unpopular with the staff because they are uncertain about how the period should be occupied, and in some it has been abandoned. It is not surprising that teachers who have had no special training for this role should find it taxing. What is so often missing is a structure of support for the tutors, and means of feeding to them ideas that can form a context for the pastoral activities, or of supporting them when faced with problems of personalities or approach.

There is great potential for creative experience in the pastoral work of the school. The tutor may readily learn some simple techniques for initiating discussion and group action (which will also flow into his approach to teaching) and for nurturing a supportive atmosphere which has its own therapeutic value. He can also be enabled to spot the social needs that require deeper attention. Above all we need to establish a sense of team work amongst the tutors so that they can offer support to one another. As a member of this team the group worker or the teacher who has acquired group work skills has a distinctive contribution to make. He can help the team to see some of the deeper implications of what is taking place in the groups, and can help to feed the pastoral groups with appropriate topics which may serve as suitable contexts for their meetings. He may also be able to work with special groups of young people referred to him by the other tutors.

School organisation

Heads and staffs of schools are having to take decisions about what kinds of groups they should bring together for teaching or pastoral purposes, often without the benefit of any clear rationale to guide their choice. For example, what weight are they to give, when forming these groups, to the natural friendships of the pupils? And what kind of pastoral structure should they adopt? Is it to be vertical (in, say, houses and even house groups consisting of representatives of all ages), or is it to be horizontal (drawing from a single age band)? And what, in terms of the relationships of the people concerned, are the pros and cons of groups of mixed ability?

The factors to be taken into account are complex. Consider, for example, the interplay of the various kinds of relationships: friendship, task, leadership and authority. The overlapping of these relationships carry both supportive and conflicting elements. As a member of a team faced by this kind of decision the group worker has much to contribute, both in the rationale upon which the decision may be based and in the means of testing the effects of the decisions taken. He may also be able to help with some of the major group influences at work in the school—for example, with attitudes that affect whole sections of the school. Fashions may invade the school, almost like epidemics, such as absenteeism and truancy, vandalism, scapegoating and even shop-lifting. These are all bound up with group pressures and group support.

It is important that, in school, we should be able to view objectively the total structure of initiative, responsibility and leadership, which in turn is bound up with the pattern of communication and consultation. The nature of consultation is widely misunderstood, and what is called consultation is often a very thin cloak over stark direction. On the other side of the coin there is often a rather precious insistence on the autonomy of the teacher in the classroom, which can mean that everyone works as a secret society. It is all part of an authoritarian tradition that prevents our helping one another. An enquiry from a senior about one's work is so often seen as interference and adverse criticism by him. This is the antithesis of relationships in group work, and teachers who have had experience of group work soon begin to question the lack of mutual help that can arise from the traditional situation.

There is rarely an objective examination of the purpose and effect of the authority structure in the schools. For example, what is the purpose of any specific prefect system? Is it to carry authority passed down from the establishment, or is it to represent the concern and identification of the pupils with their school? Sometimes this kind of question has just not been asked; in other cases, where certain objects are clearly held, the structure in no way measures up to the objectives. The group worker has the kind of technical insights and the methods that facilitate the examination of this kind of issue.

Teaching methods

There is a growing awareness of the possibility of using group forces to support work in the classroom, and in particular by working through small groups within the larger class.[1] There are a number of elements common to this kind of approach and to group work. For example, a teacher wishing to capitalise on group forces must find ways of encouraging groups to assume responsibility for their own programmes of work, and to nurture a supportive atmosphere both in small working groups and in the corporate group. There is often a combination of work in small groups with the stimulus and cross-fertilisation to be derived from sharing experiences in the corporate group. How are we to structure all this? Should we arrange for a formal structure of leadership in the small groups and of representation in the larger group, or is it better to allow an informal structure to have sway? There is even more in common between the use of discovery methods in teaching and informal group work, for discovery methods may be very similar in many ways to action research.

The skills of the group worker may also enrich team teaching, which may involve working flexibly through groups of various sizes.[2] The relationship between the class or set as a smaller unit and the corporate group will need to give each group its own standing, so that they have a stake in the organisation of the corporate activity. The corporate activities in turn require special thought in order that impetus and the commitment of everybody concerned should not be lost. And the whole process may be intensified by some of the techniques described above.

The 'team' aspect of the undertaking is not always thought through or exploited to the full. By the team is often meant the group of teachers involved, but the team should also include the young people. It is possible to enlist their support through some self-determination at small group level, and by the small groups sending representatives to a consultative body that will share with the staff any responsibilities that are within their competence.

[1] Kaye, B. and Rogers, I. (1968) *Group Work in Secondary Schools*. London: Oxford University Press.
Abercrombie, M. L. J. (1970) *Aims and Techniques of Group Teaching*. London: Society for Research into Higher Education.
[2] Warwick, D. (1971) *Team Teaching*. London: University of London Press.

Throughout this kind of work there is a shortening of distance between staff and pupils, which for many will mean new kinds of relationships. Some teachers find this difficult to take, and means must be found to help them to acclimatise themselves to new situations. The support of the staff team for one another as a tutorial group can help a great deal in this respect.

Personnel

What kind of worker, it may be asked, is going to do this type of work in school? Although the ordinary class or subject teacher will inevitably be involved in coping with group situations, it is most unlikely that more than a minority would be able or willing to work at the depth indicated in this book. The school staff may best be seen as a team, and there is a place for the specialist in group work as there is for the counsellor, the housemaster, or the head of the subject department.

There are already many hundreds of appointments of youth tutors, teacher/youth workers, and others who span the school and informal youth work. Group work is a basic skill of the youth worker, and if he knows his job he has a lot to offer to the school, not just as another teacher but as a specialist in group work and group dynamics. There are more than fifty colleges of education and university education departments offering a combined training in teaching and youth work, and providing a stream of recruits to the teaching profession who could offer group work as one of their skills.

In many schools special appointments of heads of house or heads of years have been established specifically to improve the quality of pastoral work in the school. These are key posts to which the skills of group work are appropriate, and it is very important that those who aspire to such posts should train themselves in this field. It is interesting that in various parts of the country many are seeking this kind of training on advanced courses which carry an emphasis on the dynamics of groups or which bridge the school and youth work.

Some sources for informal group work in school

CAVE, R. G. and O'MALLEY, R. (1967) *Education for Personal Responsibility*. London: Ward Lock Educational.

Connexions series. Harmondsworth: Penguin Books.

Education Today series. Harlow: Longman Group.

HACKER, ROSE. (1966) *Telling the Teenagers*. London: Deutsch.

HARRIS, A. (1968) *Questions about Living*. London: Hutchinson Educational.

HEMMING, J. (1967) *Problems of Adolescent Girls*. London: Heinemann Educational.

INGLEBY, A. (1961) *Learning to Love*. London: Robert Hale.

Looking Ahead series. Harlow: Longman Group.

Schools Council Working Papers, especially 17 *Community Service and the Curriculum* (1968). London: HMSO.

Schools Council *Humanities for the Young School Leaver* series: *an approach through classics* (1967) and *an approach through English* (1968). London: HMSO.

an approach through history (1969) and *an approach through religious education* (1969). London: Evans/Methuen Educational.

Social Education Working Papers. Nottingham: University of Nottingham School of Education.

WILSON, J. et al. (1968) *Introduction to Moral Education*. Harmondsworth: Penguin Books.

CHAPTER TEN

Group work and the wider community

Coping with outside restraints

The emphasis of this book has been on reaching the individual young person through groups of peers. Most older adolescents spend a very large part of their lives with their peers, as they loosen their connections with their families and other settled community groups. Thus the peer group is used both as a vehicle for personal development, and as a framework of support for the youngster coping with pressures outside the group. In this context, we must include in 'support' helping the adolescent to prepare his own strategies to meet these situations. In this respect group work with younger children may need a different orientation.

When these outside pressures represent a major factor in the life of a youngster, they may seriously limit what can be accomplished within the peer group setting, and the worker must ask himself whether he must not reach out to those outside restraints. We have already looked at an example of this in the young people who are in conflict with school. We may be able to offer some compensatory experience away from the source of the conflict, but its real resolution, or any restitution for a hurt that has been inflicted, should ultimately be tackled at the source of the conflict.

Facing himself with this problem, the worker will need to consider the extent to which he should involve young people in helping to change the situations in which they are entangled. It is unlikely that many of them will be able, without help, to change difficult situations that involve their seniors in age or authority. It is much more likely that the group worker will need to warm up the dialogue by himself engaging each of the parties before the young person will be in a strong enough position to play his part. This can be a delicate operation for the group worker. Take as an example the difficulties experienced by young people at school: it is tricky enough for the worker who is rubbing shoulders with the staff as a member of the same team; the group worker who must approach the school from outside can easily be seen as an alien and interfering body.

The dialogue

I should like to distinguish between a dialogue and confrontation. In a confrontation the parties tend to determine their position before a meeting takes place and wish only to demolish the other person's case, or even to demolish him personally. A dialogue implies that each party enters a meeting with the intention of making clear his own position, but at the same time wishing to understand the other person's point of view. Before a dialogue can be said to have taken place, both parties—and in particular the senior party if there is a difference in status—must have been seen as open to change. Similarly, when teaching through a dialogue, the teacher must himself be open to the influence of his pupils and be prepared to learn from them. An absence of this kind of openness will show the approach through a dialogue to have been a pretence, and may rapidly lead to a confrontation.

There are therefore several prerequisites to a dialogue. The channels of communication must be open. This does not mean only that the people concerned are prepared to engage in a conversation, but also that any topic relevant to the discussion on hand will be seen as legitimate. Since the difficulties are sometimes being caused by the avoidance of prohibited areas of conversation, this is a step that may need considerable preparation. Many of the conflicts with parents are on the surface about one thing (for example, the time of returning home at night), whereas at root they may be about another (the parents' unspoken anxiety about the youngster's sexual behaviour). As a result of long restraints certain areas of conversation may become virtually outlawed. It is often very difficult for the youngster to approach these subjects unaided, and even if he were to do so, he might face an unreasoning rebuff from the senior partner, who is also in difficulties with the same topic. In order to clear such impediment to the growth of the youngster, it may be necessary for the worker to open up new areas of communication with both the parties.

It is rare that the need for change is in one of the parties only, and the worker is in danger of seeing a wrong perspective if he hears only the youngster's side of the question. He may find that the situation seems exactly the opposite to, say, the parent or the teacher. Sometimes it is only necessary for the worker to act as a third party in order to lead a conversation to a more objective examination of hitherto unspoken areas of concern. But only too often there has been a breakdown in communication, and possibly serious confrontation and conflict. In these cases it may be necessary for the worker to see each party separately several times, encouraging them to examine their own position and to consider factors that they may have ignored. Only when he considers that there is sufficient common ground between the parties will he encourage them to enter into a dialogue, probably with him as a third party.

The burden that some young people carry may be so severe and intractable that little can be done to offer immediate amelioration, and the best that can be offered by the group is to help the youngster to bear his difficulties.[1] Often, troubles are compounded. Unsatisfactory conditions at home may be a contributory cause to mischief at school, with the result that the youngster who most needs support and understanding draws the wrath of the school upon him. This may serve to reinforce the youngster's feelings about authority. Or a stereotyped personal role that has its roots in the family may be reinforced by the youngster's peers, or even his teachers. In this way an unhelpful life style may become settled unless someone intervenes before the youngster reaches adult status. Sometimes the youth worker is forced to add his weight to the confirmation of social disability, when he finds it necessary to exclude troublesome youngsters from his club in order to preserve its usefulness to the majority. In fact he may be responding to the youngster's tendency to seek rejection.

[1] Clegg, A. and Megson, B. (1968) *Children in Distress*. Harmondsworth: Penguin Books.
Schools Council (1970) Working Paper 27, '*Cross'd with Adversity*'. London: Evans/Methuen Educational.

Reaching the family

All the time the worker will be having to judge what is within his influence and what is not. He will meet youngters who face appalling problems at home, arising, for example, from the drunkenness of the father, or the fickleness or near prostitution of the mother. Many such situations are beyond the marginal influence open to most workers concerned primarily with adolescents, and he must look to the local social services or the family service unit if one exists, to help with this kind of situation. At the other end of the scale some of the conflicts with parents that so overwhelm young people may arise almost entirely out of a lack of communication, and very often express the concern—perhaps the over-concern—of the parents for the youngster. In many of these cases the group worker can offer very considerable help by enabling communication to deepen.

We first developed informal group work in the setting of youth work, and we accepted the prevailing attitudes amongst youth workers that young people would resist and resent any contacts between the worker and his parents. We now see this as one of our untested preconceptions, and as part of the same timidity that held us back from making direct contacts with young people. As the work progressed and individual workers have had occasion to make contact with the homes of young people, they have found that they have been warmly received by most parents, and the young people also seemed pleased that the workers had taken this amount of interest and trouble. The reluctance of the workers to take this step has been in part as a result of their own fear of rejection.

Naturally, any visits to parents about a topic under discussion with the youngster would be by agreement with that youngster, but a number of workers first learnt about the welcome that awaited them when they visited several homes in order to leave urgent messages or for some other quite neutral purpose. A worker concerned with a group of girls at school, whose parents were thought to be antagonistic to the school and unhelpful to the youngsters, found it necessary to visit more homes than she had intended in order not to disappoint some of the youngsters who wanted their parents to be visited also. She certainly did not find the parents 'antagonistic': diffident would have been a much better description. Teachers rarely test their assertion that parents who do not attend open days and other school occasions are those who lack interest in their children. We can under-estimate the effect of the parents' feelings towards people in authority, their own memories of school, or merely their general confusion or timidity.

Often we find that the youngster has completely misjudged the parents' position. This is illustrated by the case of a boy who reported serious hostility towards him by his father. When the worker called to deliver a message, the father immediately engaged the worker in a wider conversation and expressed his concern for the boy, adding, 'You must find him a handful down at the club.' The worker was able to reply that on the contrary they found him cooperative and an interesting character. That single visit, together with an immediate discussion with the youngster, was enough to change the course of events by opening up a new level of conversation between the boy and his parents. It is sometimes possible to bring the youngster to see that his parents also need help; parents may have considerable adjustments to make as their children grow older and change their position in the family. As he grows in stature through helping other members of the group, and possibly people outside the group through a programme of action research and community service, he may soon be ready to cope with his own situation at home in a helpful and creative way. In approaching this situation, he may be helped deliberately by the group, who may discuss with him events at home as they occur, explore their real meaning through socio-drama, and help him to prepare his next step through role-play. Some young people are more mature or more socially able than their parents.

If there are several members of the group who are ill at ease at home, this may be made the central context of the group. We have found that it can be one of the norms of some groups that they *must* be seen as in conflict with their families, which can be dealt with like any other normative change. In other cases, in which the main trouble has been a lack of communication rather than unhelpful personalities in the parents, the group has arranged interesting meetings with parents. For example, some groups have visited each home in turn, and discussed relationships between the generations with the parents in their own homes. Other groups have led into parents' conventions through action research; in some cases the convention has been open to young people outside their own immediate group.

G

Sometimes difficulties at home are never discussed by a natural friendship group in spite of their being a major pre-occupation of most of the members. It is as if the subject were taboo, in case it should open a floodgate of emotion that the members of the group would not be able to control. It may be no accident that the girl who was being scapegoated by one such group had a particularly difficult home situation: it was as if, through her, they were holding the whole subject at bay. In this kind of case, unless the worker's diagnosis is good and rapid the conspiracy of silence may prevent his perceiving one of the group's most urgent needs. It is the presence of the worker, as an objective third party inducing a supportive and controlled situation, that makes possible the incursion into areas of life that are highly charged emotionally.

The neighbourhood

A number of groups who have been led to expressing their compassion for people less fortunate than themselves, or in other ways have taken an active and constructive interest in the community, have wanted to to do all this outside their immediate neighbourhood. In most cases this has been because their action would be uncharacteristic of their neighbourhood, and they feared that they would lose face if they behaved in inappropriate ways. They are merely revealing how much of their life is governed by the prevailing—possibly anti-social—normative controls of the neighbourhood.

When this situation obtains, the work within a small peer group is likely to be inhibited by the surrounding climate; in fact the members of the group may well behave differently when they are with the worker from the way they behave when at large in their neighbourhood. When viewing what may seem to us to be a lack of adjustment, it is important to distinguish between personal maladjustment and the effects of deviant cultures. Some delinquency arises from social ineptitude, but some of it stems from all too apt an adjustment to unhelpful norms, such as hostility to school, irresponsibility, vandalism, violence, and fixed and violent feelings towards authority. In certain circumstances, 'successful' group work could lead to an alienation from the surrounding peer culture—and from the adult culture also in some cases.

The group worker may feel daunted when faced by serious problems that emanate from outside the group as well as by the personal problems of the members of the group. Major neighbourhood changes may need the concerted action of the social agencies in the area, and particularly of the school. It may have been a disadvantage in this respect that many smaller neighbourhood secondary schools have been replaced by larger schools drawing from a very wide area without a sense of neighbourhood.

The group worker may have to be satisfied with small gains, but if he wishes to ease unhelpful community pressures on his group of young people and to make a contribution to changes in neighbourhood patterns of behaviour, he must have these two objectives clearly before him. Our experience would suggest that the case is not as hopeless as it would first appear and, seen in long term, youngsters may be prepared to act as agents of change in their own locality. For example, on a totally working-class council house estate, almost devoid of indigenous leadership, an important object was to nurture the potential leadership of the members of the group. This began as joint action and initiative in the group, but was soon fed into initiating action for other people. A group involved in action research somewhat surprised themselves by gaining the attention of several of the elders of their district, and at this point began to take seriously their own capacity for social action.

If the work is taking place within a youth club or other larger institution, there may be an arena for practising leadership and social action readily at hand. It is really most impressive when one sees an erstwhile violent gang first moderate their own behaviour, and ultimately reach out to influence and occupy younger children who are just reaching the stage of serious vandalism. Although it may take time for individual youngsters to pass through a series of stages on their way to responsible attitudes and a capacity to serve others, it is possible that a group may in a single step decide that they wish to go in this way, and that they will prepare themselves for responsible leadership amongst their own peers and in the community at large.

The community school

The school is caught up in the same kind of pattern of social influences, and what can be achieved in school is influenced by the restraints emanating from the expectations of the community around it. This is not restricted to the overt demands and expressions of opinion outside the school, for the unconscious expectancies brought into the school by the pupils are even more powerful. In this sense the community and its influence is continually with the school.

There has been a rapid growth of the concept of the community school. This is often seen as offering the facilities of the school to the surrounding community. The school may become a centre for further education and the kinds of activities offered in many districts for evening centres may also be brought into day-time programmes by using special accommodation made available for this purpose. In this way members of the adult community become accustomed to moving in and out of the school quite naturally and the points of interaction established in this way may be used for an ever-growing dialogue between the school and the local population. But if the community school is to have its full sway it must be seen in a broader context than this.[1]

The school is the only social agency that is readily in touch with most of the community, and in particular with families having children of school age within them. No other social service has such an opportunity for social education amongst the normal community. The traditional vehicle for social education has been and still is the family, and yet so much in modern life weakens the position of the parent. Think, for example, of the dilemma being experienced by parents in their relationships with their older children. Many parents are at a disadvantage in a number of ways, for the experience of young people has taken them into areas of which their parents have had little or no experience themselves. If parents in this position are to continue to have influence with their children they will need considerable help from the school, partly in terms of keeping up to date with trends in education—not that they would need to know everything that the youngster is learning, but they would at least need to know about it—but also in supporting their determination to play their full part as a parent.

[1] Carr, D. (1973) 'A role for the Community School'. *Youth in Society*, November/December 1973 (pages 6-10).
Bessey, G. (1968) 'The Community School'. *R.I.B.A. Journal*, August 1968 (pages 364-8).

The way that a parent is expected to behave towards his or her child will not be a matter of personal judgement alone: it will be subject to the prevailing climate in the surrounding community. The school is inevitably the potent force in this local climate and even the insular attitudes that characterise some schools speak eloquently in this respect. It is not enough to put our faith in the occasional meetings of Parent/Teacher Associations, and to complain that the parents we most wish to see do not come along. The school will need to take a much more dynamic part in all this, and something more akin to what is described as the techniques of group work will be appropriate to the role of the school in the community.

Within a community of workers

It is vital that the group worker should keep at the forefront of his mind that he is only one of a number of workers who will be offering a personal service within his neighbourhood. He should make himself familiar with the other services that are available, and seek also a working relationship with the actual workers involved. Above all, the group worker should recognise the limitations in what he can offer through group work. His contact with other workers will need to be specific as well as general when coping with a young person whom another worker might help or with whom he may already be in contact. It is important that the group worker should see himself as a member of a team, and in this respect he will reach out both to the other social services and to the school. In some ways he can help to maintain contact between the school and the social workers in the district.

Group work, as an approach to different kinds of problems, may also be part of the skill of a number of social workers. Group work is the basic skill of the youth worker, and has relevance to the school, as has already been suggested. It also has a valuable contribution to make to probation work, child care, the family services and mental health as group therapy. It is applicable to work with both young and old.

Training for social work has tended to be concentrated on case work, but many of the situations faced by social workers are so bound up with personal relationships and group controls that only a limited amount of help can be offered through individual case work. For example, it is very difficult to offer a young person the kind of experience he needs to help him in his skill in relating to his peers through a one-to-one relationship with an adult case worker. The skills of group work are essential to the social worker in some of the situations he faces. An obvious example of this is in the work of the probation officer. If the probation officer were to be really 'successful' with some of his clients, he could easily alienate them from their normal social containment with their peers. In fact, there is not much likelihood of this happening.

Conversely, it is impossible to approach group work in the style suggested in this book without certain skills in case work and counselling. Some of the development of individual young people is helped along by interviews and intimate conversation, and in continuing personal contact away from the whole group. Community development is another related but discrete field of work.[1] The community development worker is more concerned with the broad organisational structure within which all groups can operate creatively. Everything he attempts is conditioned by the dynamics of the groups around him, and some skill in group work is valuable to him. But he is not usually a group worker in the more intimate sense of seeing the personal development of individual people as the basic criteria for the group's activity.

It is probably unrealistic to see the functions of the case worker, group worker and community development worker vested in a single person, although they will need to be very much aware of one another's work and to borrow one another's skills. Personality and temperament will affect the sphere of work to which individuals will gravitate. The crucial point is that these three kinds of worker should see themselves as a team.

Their functions overlap. The immediate personal support required by an individual at a time of crisis is pre-eminently in the field of the case worker, but he will also be concerned with personal development, particularly through developmental counselling. The group worker's main fields of work are personality development at one end, through social education to group activity and liberal education at the other. He is less concerned with crisis work and community organisation, though both of

---

[1] Gulbenkian Report (ed.) (1968) *Community Work and Social Change.* London: Longmans Green.
Leaper, R. (1971) *Community Work.* London: National Council of Social Service.

these may be elements in some of his work. The community development worker is primarily concerned with community organisation, though social and liberal education will be an essential ingredient of much of his work. The continuing health of our communities calls for service on a broad front, which will be facilitated by the close collaboration of educationists and social workers.

Appendices

Appendix 1a—Group enquiry I

Name ....

Group ....

1 Who are the members of the group?

2 What holds the group together?

3 What does the group do?

4 Has the group a routine?

    (*a*) What happens on a typical evening?

(*b*) What happened?

	Where did you meet?	What happened?
Monday		
Tuesday		
Wednesday		
Thursday		
Friday		
Saturday afternoon		
Saturday evening		
Sunday morning		
Sunday afternoon		
Sunday evening		

(*c*) Was last week typical?

5 Did everyone turn up each time?

6 Are there times when you expect everyone to be there?

7 If one of the group didn't turn up, then we . . .

8 Do you all wear similar clothes?

9 If so, why?

10 I would be in trouble with the group if I were to . . .

11 What would they do?

12 When you are away from the group do you ever:
    (*a*) behave differently?

    How?

    (*b*) do different things?

    What kind of things?

Appendix 1b—Group enquiry II

Name ....

Group ....

1   I like it best when the group . . .

2   I don't like it when the group . . .

3   The group are all pleased when . . .

4   The group gets angry when . . .

    What do they do about it?

5   The most daring thing we do as a group is to . . .

6   When we come across other groups of our own age, for
    example . . .

    we . . .

7   If there is chance of trouble we . . .

8   As we move about the town we . . .

9   If any of our group damaged something, for example . . .

    we . . .

10   When we are/were at school we . . .

11   If any members of our group played truant the rest of us would . . .

12   To us, hard work at school was . . .

13   We didn't like teachers who . . .

14   At work we would expect the members of our group to . . .

15   When we meet an adult, say . . .

we . . .

16   The group would expect me to . . .

. . . my parents.

17   When the police are about we . . .

18   When the group come across any boys/girls (members of the opposite sex) we . . .

19   If a member of the group started getting serious about a boy/girl the rest of us would . . .

20   If I went out with a boy/girl the group would expect me to . . .

Appendix 1c—Group enquiry III

Name ....

Group ....

1   What do you talk about in the group?

2   Do you talk about:
   (*a*)   clothes/make-up?
   (*b*)   sport or some other activities?
          What activities?
   (*c*)   school or work?
   (*d*)   home and parents?
   (*e*)   boy friends or girl friends?
   (*f*)   sex?
   (*g*)   religion?
   (*h*)   politics?
   (*i*)   what else?

3   The group would *not* like me to talk to them about . . .

4   The group wouldn't like it if I didn't tell them about . . .

5   Would you talk to the group about things that were going badly:
   (*a*)   at school or work?
   (*b*)   at home?
   (*c*)   with your boy-friend or girl-friend?

6   Do you ever do anything that you would not like the group to know about?

       What kind of things?

7 When you are alone with certain members of the group, do you talk about things that you would not tell the group as a whole?

With.. I talk about . . .

With.. I talk about . . .

With.. I talk about . . .

8 Do members of the group ever talk about how they feel about themselves?

What kind of feelings?

Appendix 1d—Group enquiry IV

Name ....

Group ....

1 Do any members of the group behave in a special way of their own?

Name   *Special behaviour*

2 Do any of the members do anything special *for* the group?

Name   *Special behaviour*

3 How would you rate the contribution, to the group, of each member in:

(*a*) suggesting things to do.
(*b*) getting things done.
(*c*) keeping the peace.
(*d*) leading the group.
(*e*) being a disruptive influence in the group.
(*f*) leading the fun.

Award 1 to 5 marks for each (1 = low, 5 = high).

Name	(a)	(b)	(c)	(d)	(e)	(f)

4 How do you rate yourself in this group?

5 Are you a member of other situations or groups? How do you rate yourself in those other groups?

Situation or group	(a)	(b)	(c)	(d)	(e)	(f)

6 If the group was going to do something:

(a) who would be most likely to have suggested it?

(b) how would it be decided?

(*c*) how would you get to know?

(*d*) who do you think would be the best person to organise it?

(*e*) who would actually organise it?

7 If you wanted the group to do something:
   (*a*) to whom would you look as an ally?

   (*b*) who would be most likely to be able to stop it if he wanted to?

   (*c*) who could persuade the others if he wanted to?

The purpose of self-description is to help the subject's self-searching and our diagnosis. The emphasis is on self-description rather than evaluation. It is not just something that the subject puts on paper, but rather an opportunity to explore inside himself in the hope that it will help him to determine the kinds of modification he would like to make in his own behaviour. Ideally we would wish to create a situation where he shares this self-discovery with his colleagues in the group.

The manner in which the self-description is approached is as important as the format of questioning. For example, a widely ranging discussion about self-feelings and personal behaviour will produce something quite different from a more mechanical response to a series of questions. Sometimes a combination of the two approaches is possible, with a general discussion in a group setting preceding a response to each question in turn.

A *pro forma* for self-description is in the last resort a list of qualities, of behaviours and personal feelings. Sometimes an attempt is made to separate behaviour from feelings, and in other cases the self description *pro forma* is built on a list of personality traits. The individual worker will need to make up his mind what elements he needs to bring into the discussion, first, in order to enable the people with whom he is working to express themselves in ways that will be helpful to them, and second, to suit the general style of work taking place.

Form A has been evolved from themes that have recurred in our work with young people, and, with adults too. The approach is open-ended, which not only gives freedom to the respondent, but also demands considerable thought. But for the exercise to be carried through successfully, the subject will need to be fairly articulate, and capable of perceiving his own feelings and behaviour.

Form B is a rather simpler, self-rating scale. When using self-rating scales we have found that the range of two or three alternatives—for example, like me, not like me, do not know—is somewhat limiting. We have found that a five-point scale is often more satisfactory. Form B is such a framework, appropriate for some groups of young people.

We have found in general that although this rather more mechanical format is easier to use and to respond to, its value to the respondent is not always as great as a more open-ended approach that demands greater effort and thought. The worker needs to judge the level of sophistication of the group with whom he is working and plan his approach accordingly, not forgetting that raising the level of sophistication is one of the purposes of his work with them.

Kelly suggests, as an alternative approach, a descriptive character sketch written in prose.[1] The subject is invited to write a letter to a friend about himself in the third person, as if he were a second friend. The reader may feel that this kind of approach is much more appropriate to well-educated subjects attending psychiatric sessions than to most of the groups he meets. But this approach has much to offer in some school situations, where a character sketch would not be out of place as a normal piece of prose writing.

Several forms of self-concept description or inventory have been developed,[2] and self-concept tests have been used for evaluative purposes.[3] Self-concept tests are often administered in two forms, first for the actual self, and second for the ideal self.[4] Form B can be used in this way.

[1] Kelly, G. (1955) *The Psychology of Personal Constructs*. New York: Norton. (Especially Chapter 7—The Analysis of Self-Characterisation; Chapter 8—Fixed-Role Therapy.)
See also Bannister, D. and Fransella, F. (1971) *Inquiring Man*. Harmondsworth: Penguin Books. (Especially pages 78–83.)
[2] Purkey, W. W. (1968) *The Search for Self: Evaluating Student Self-Concepts*. Research Bulletin, No. 2. Florida Educational Research and Development Council.
[3] Payne, J., Drummond, A. W. and Lunghi, M. (1970) 'Changes in Self Concepts of School Leavers who participated in an Arctic Expedition.' *British Journal of Educational Psychology*, Vol. 40, Part 2, 211–15.
[4] For a general view of self-concept studies see Wylie, R. C. (1961) *The Self Concept*. Lincoln, Nebr.: University of Nebraska Press.

Form C is included as an illustration of the way in which a self-description may be adapted to specific purposes, in this case as part of some in-service training for full-time youth workers.

Form A: Self-description

1 What is my level of self-esteem (feelings of personal worth, sense of inferiority)?

2 How shy or reserved am I? How outgoing or daring in contact with people?

3 How self-reliant am I (self sufficient—as distinct from reserved, dependent)?

4 Am I reliable (trustworthy, honest, evasive)?

5 Am I persistent and consistent or fickle and restless?

6 Am I flexible, spontaneous, rigid, inhibited?

7 How do I take uncertainty?

8 Have I resilience to criticism and hostility? How do I respond?

9 How do I feel when I am rejected, or suspect that I might be rejected?

10 How dominant or submissive am I?

11   How emotional am I? And what kind of emotion pre-
     dominates (aggressive, impulsive, demanding, even-tempered,
     phlegmatic)?

12   Am I sensitive to others (in the sense of distinguishing what
     others are feeling and thinking)?

13   Have I compassion and sympathy for others?

14   Friendship:

     (*a*) Do I find friendship-forming easy or difficult?

     (*b*) Am I content with my circle of friends?

     (*c*) How far do I/can I let friends into my intimate self?

15   How do I operate in groups?

     (*a*) Do I find myself acceptable/unacceptable to other
            people? And in what ways?

     (*b*) What kind of role do I take in groups?

     (*c*) Is it a recurring role? How flexible is it?

Form B: Self-description—Inventory

	Very much like me	Like me	Neutral Doubtful	Not like me	Not at all like me
1 I feel shy when I meet new people.					
2 I am frightened that people will find out too much about what I am like.					
3 I feel that I am a nice person to know.					
4 I often feel that I am a failure.					
5 I want to be liked.					
6 I keep myself to myself.					
7 I am honest and trustworthy.					
8 My friends can depend upon me.					
9 I will stick to something until I have finished it.					
10 I'm very changeable.					
11 I always stick to what I say, no matter whether I am right or wrong.					
12 When I come up against an obstacle I try another way round it.					
13 I find it difficult to let myself go.					
14 I can't stand uncertainty.					
15 I get angry when people criticise me.					
16 When someone threatens me I become frightened.					

	Very much like me	Like me	Neutral Doubtful	Not like me	Not at all like me
17 When someone is angry with me I am immediately angry with him.					
18 I am disturbed if people leave me out of things.					
19 I like to lead rather than to follow.					
20 I tend to be moody.					
21 I can usually sense what people are feeling.					
22 I am very stirred when I see other people unhappy or in personal difficulty.					
23 I make friends easily.					
24 I always like to have a lot of people around me.					
25 I always behave in certain ways when I am with a group.					

Form C: Self-description for full-time youth workers

1 How easy or difficult do I find it to open up conversation with members of staff about:

(a) daily tasks to be undertaken?

(b) the way they perform their tasks?

(c) their more personal feelings about what they are attempting?

2 Do I fear rejection; am I prepared to risk rejection of or opposition to what I propose?

3 How conscious am I of the possibility of criticism (spoken or unspoken) of me?

   Does the fear of criticism in any way inhibit my action or approach?

4 How far do I need the approbation of certain members of staff, or can I go my own way?

5 Do I expect other people to accept what I say?

6 How do I respond to a crisis—for example, do I flap?

7 Can I get stuck in to a difficult or prickly job, or do I dither?

8 How resilient am I when things are difficult—can I keep pressing forward when others are doubting?

9 What is my general level of persistence?

10 How do I feel about myself; for example:
   (*a*) am I a successful person, or a failure?

   (*b*) am I a likeable person?

   (*c*) am I an efficient person?

   (*d*) am I an easy person to get on with?

11 What kind of person am I?

Index